Rabies Virus at the Beginning of 21st Century

Edited by Sergey Tkachev

Published in London, United Kingdom

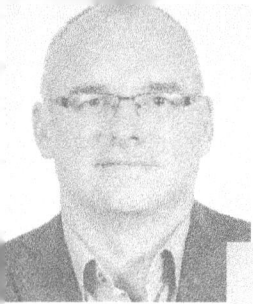
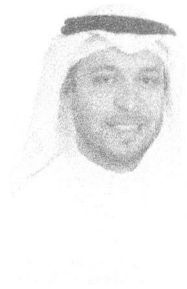
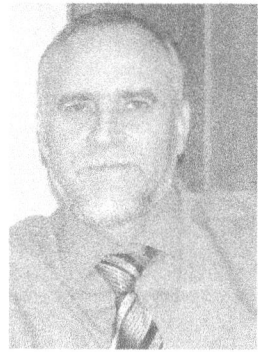
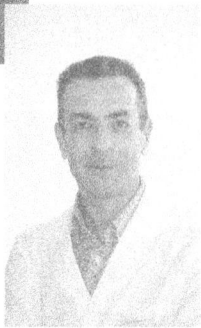
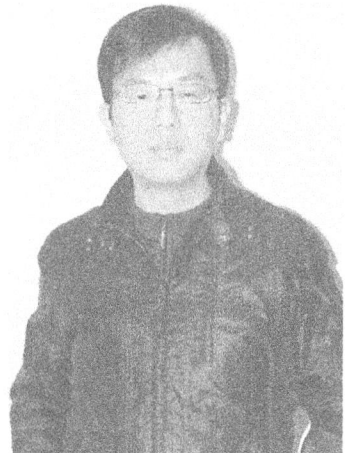
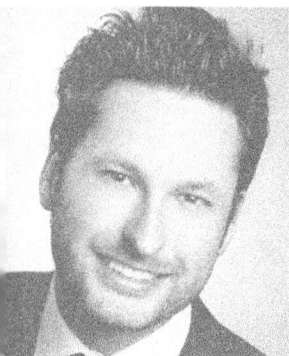
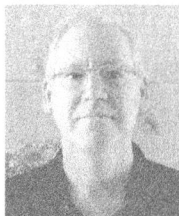

IntechOpen

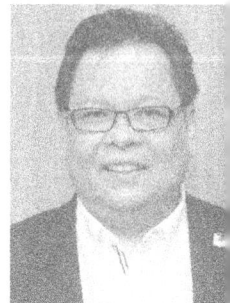
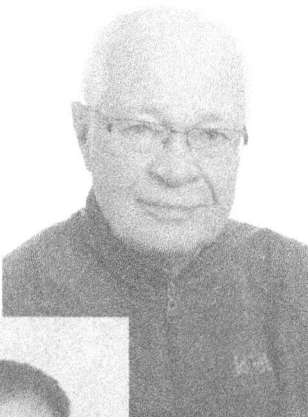
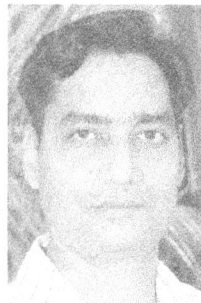
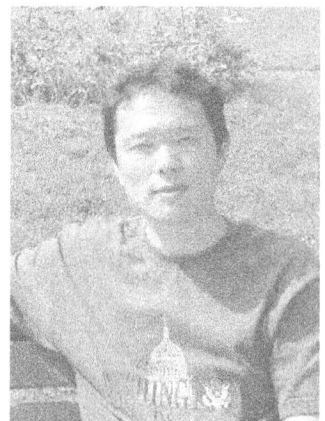
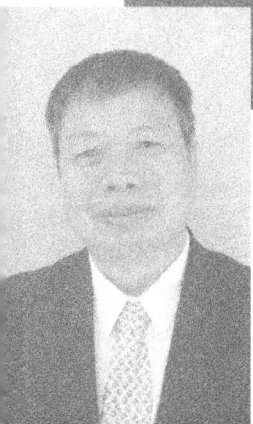
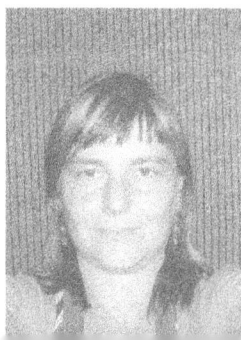

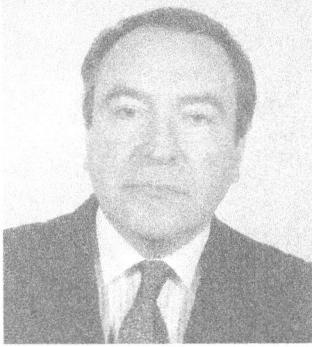

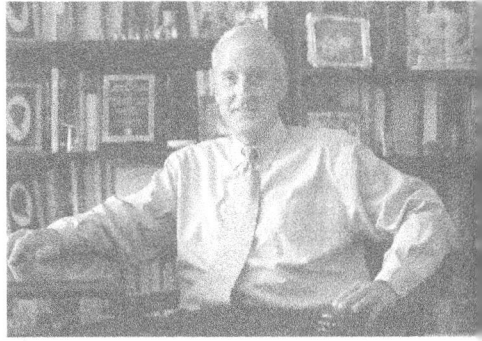

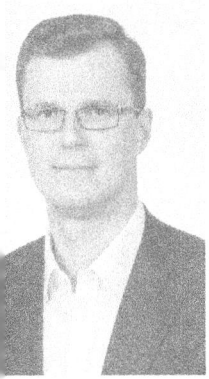

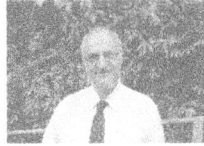

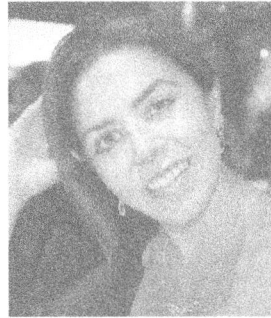

Supporting open minds since 2005

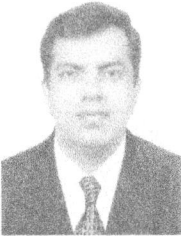

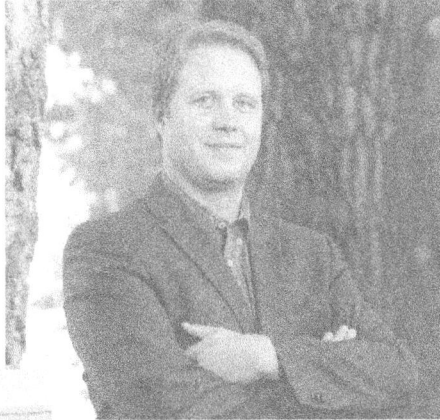

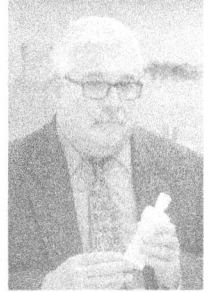

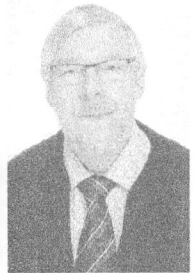

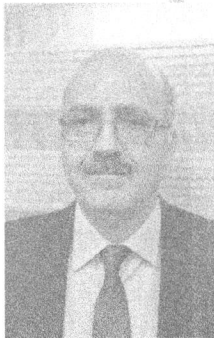

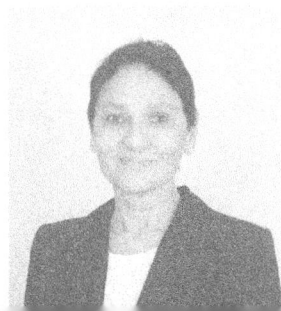

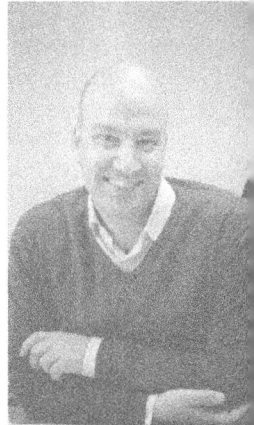

Rabies Virus at the Beginning of 21st Century
http://dx.doi.org/10.5772/intechopen.80154
Edited by Sergey Tkachev

Contributors
Roland Suluku, Benjamin Emikpe, Abu Macavoray, Moinina Nelphson Kallon, Namera Thahaby, Afzal Hoque Akand, Shabeer Ahmed Hamdani, Abdul Hai Bhat, Mudasir Ali Rather, Abdelmalik I. Khalafalla, Yahia H. Ali, Richard Lathe, Marie-Paule Kieny, Sean M. Richards, Samantha Sweck, Jaida Hopkins, Sergey Tkachev

Notice
Statements and opinions expressed in the chapters are these of the individual contributors and not necessarily those of the editors or publisher. No responsibility is accepted for the accuracy of information contained in the published chapters. The publisher assumes no responsibility for any damage or injury to persons or property arising out of the use of any materials, instructions, methods or ideas contained in the book.

First published in London, United Kingdom, 2022 by IntechOpen
IntechOpen is the global imprint of INTECHOPEN LIMITED, registered in England and Wales, registration number: 11086078, 5 Princes Gate Court, London, SW7 2QJ, United Kingdom
Printed in Croatia

British Library Cataloguing-in-Publication Data
A catalogue record for this book is available from the British Library

Additional hard and PDF copies can be obtained from orders@intechopen.com

Rabies Virus at the Beginning of 21st Century
Edited by Sergey Tkachev
p. cm.

This title is part of the Veterinary Medicine and Science Book Series, Volume 9
Topic: Animal Science
Series Editor: Rita Payan Carreira
Topic Editor: Edward Narayan

Print ISBN 978-1-83969-229-1
Online ISBN 978-1-83969-230-7
eBook (PDF) ISBN 978-1-83969-231-4
ISSN 2632-0517

We are IntechOpen,
the world's leading publisher of
Open Access books
Built by scientists, for scientists

5,800+
Open access books available

142,000+
International authors and editors

180M+
Downloads

Our authors are among the

156
Countries delivered to

Top 1%
most cited scientists

12.2%
Contributors from top 500 universities

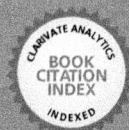

Interested in publishing with us?
Contact book.department@intechopen.com

Numbers displayed above are based on latest data collected.
For more information visit www.intechopen.com

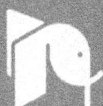

IntechOpen Book Series
Veterinary Medicine and Science
Volume 9

Aims and Scope of the Series

Paralleling similar advances in the medical field, astounding advances occurred in Veterinary Medicine and Science in recent decades. These advances have helped foster better support for animal health, more humane animal production, and a better understanding of the physiology of endangered species to improve the assisted reproductive technologies or the pathogenesis of certain diseases, where animals can be used as models for human diseases (like cancer, degenerative diseases or fertility), and even as a guarantee of public health. Bridging Human, Animal, and Environmental health, the holistic and integrative "One Health" concept intimately associates the developments within those fields, projecting its advancements into practice. This book series aims to tackle various animal-related medicine and sciences fields, providing thematic volumes consisting of high-quality significant research directed to researchers and postgraduates. It aims to give us a glimpse into the new accomplishments in the Veterinary Medicine and Science field. By addressing hot topics in veterinary sciences, we aim to gather authoritative texts within each issue of this series, providing in-depth overviews and analysis for graduates, academics, and practitioners and foreseeing a deeper understanding of the subject. Forthcoming texts, written and edited by experienced researchers from both industry and academia, will also discuss scientific challenges faced today in Veterinary Medicine and Science. In brief, we hope that books in this series will provide accessible references for those interested or working in this field and encourage learning in a range of different topics.

Meet the Series Editor

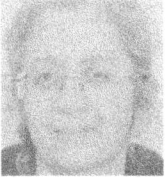

Rita Payan Carreira earned her Veterinary Degree from the Faculty of Veterinary Medicine in Lisbon, Portugal, in 1985. She obtained her Ph.D. in Veterinary Sciences from the University of Trás-os-Montes e Alto Douro, Portugal. After almost 32 years of teaching at the University of Trás-os-Montes and Alto Douro, she recently moved to the University of Évora, Department of Veterinary Medicine, where she teaches in the field of Animal Reproduction and Clinics. Her primary research areas include the molecular markers of the endometrial cycle and the embryo–maternal interaction, including oxidative stress and the reproductive physiology and disorders of sexual development, besides the molecular determinants of male and female fertility. She often supervises students preparing their master's or doctoral theses. She is also a frequent referee for various journals.

Meet the Volume Editor

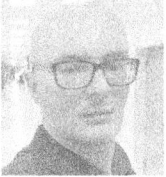

Dr. Sergey Tkachev is a senior research scientist at the Institute of Fundamental Medicine and Biology, Kazan Federal University, Russia, and at the Institute of Chemical Biology and Fundamental Medicine SB RAS, Novosibirsk, Russia. He received his Ph.D. in Molecular Biology with his thesis "Genetic variability of the tick-borne encephalitis virus in natural foci of Novosibirsk city and its suburbs." His primary field is molecular virology with research emphasis on vector-borne viruses, especially tick-borne encephalitis virus, Kemerovo virus and Omsk hemorrhagic fever virus, rabies virus, molecular genetics, biology, and epidemiology of virus pathogens.

Contents

Preface

Rabies is a zoonotic viral disease that is fatal once clinical manifestations develop. Its agent, the rabies virus (RABV), is a (-)ssRNA virus belonging to the order *Mononegavirales*, the family *Rhabdoviridae* (from the Latin word "rhabdos", meaning "rod," because representatives of this family have rod-shaped virions), and the genus *Lyssavirus* (from the name "Lyssa," an ancient Greek goddess, the personification of rabies).

Despite significant progress in fighting rabies worldwide and successful eradication programs in Western Europe, rabies remains an important public health concern, causing approximately 50,000 human cases per year. Rabies is present on every continent except Antarctica and Australia, with 95% of human deaths occurring in Asia and Africa. In almost 99% of cases, the transmission of RABV to humans occurs from domestic dogs. However, rabies can affect both domestic and wild animals and can be transmitted to humans through bites or scratches, usually through saliva.

This book summarizes current knowledge regarding RABV, its prevalence and genetic diversity, and modern approaches to its diagnosis, prevention, and treatment. It is a useful resource for scientists, doctors, and students studying the problem of rabies, conducting research, carrying out preventive measures, and providing medical care to patients.

Dr. Sergey Tkachev
Institute of Fundamental Medicine and Biology of Kazan Federal University,
Kazan, Russia

Institute of Chemical Biology and Fundamental Medicine SB RAS,
Novosibirsk, Russia

Section 1

Common Issues
of the Rabies Virus

Chapter 1

Introductory Chapter: Rabies in the 21st Century

Sergey Tkachev

1. Introduction

Rabies is known as a fatal viral infection that is most commonly spread to humans and pets through the bites, scratches, or contamination of mucous membranes with the infected saliva of an infected animal. In an infected organism, an acute progressive encephalomyelitis/encephalitis develops ultimately resulting in death.

The infection is caused by a neurotropic zoonotic virus belonging to the *Lyssavirus* genus (named after *Lyssa*, an ancient Greek goddess, the personification of rabies) of the *Rhabdoviridae* family (from the Latin *rhabdos*, meaning "rod", because the members of this family have rod-shaped virions). Currently, the *Lyssavirus* genus contains 18 virus species (https://talk.ictvonline.org/), and between them, the rabies virus is the most important one concerning its impact on public health.

2. Molecular biology of rabies virus

The rabies virus (RABV) is enveloped, bullet-shaped viruses, 180 nm in length and 75 nm wide (**Figure 1**). Virions are composed of two structural units: an

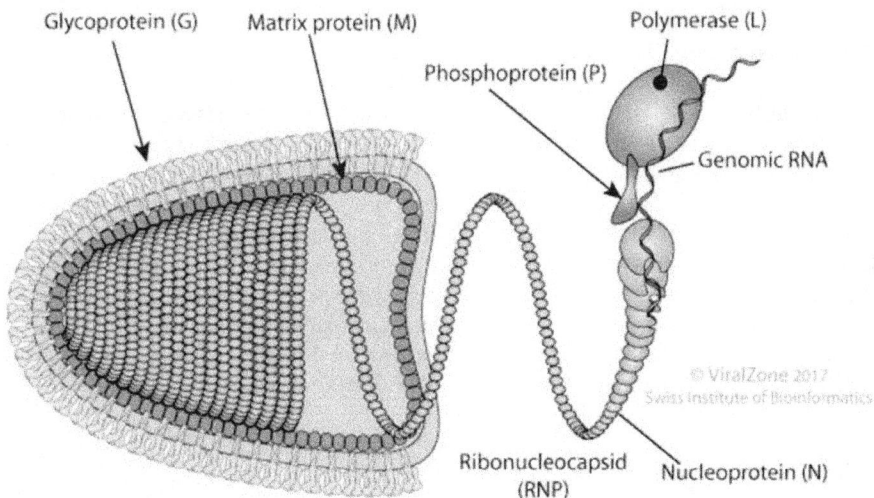

Figure 1.
The structure of the rabies virus (https://viralzone.expasy.org/22).

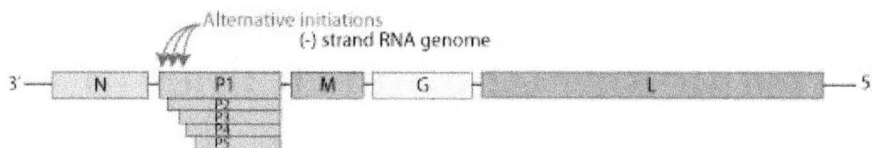

Figure 2.
Genome structure of the rabies virus (https://viralzone.expasy.org/22).

internal helical nucleocapsid (consisting of nucleoprotein N and viral genome RNA), and a lipid envelope derived from the host cytoplasmic membrane during virus budding.

RABV contains a negative-sense ssRNA genome 11.9–12.3 kb in length, encoding five protein-coding genes: N, P, M, G, and L, which are separated by intergenic regions of variable length (**Figure 2**) [1]. P gene has alternative initiation points that lead to translation of P protein and at least four additional shorter gene products [2]. At 3′- and 5′- ends of RABV genome 58 nt leader sequence, and 57–70 nt trailer is located, subsequently [3].

3. Genetic diversity of rabies virus

Currently, phylogenetic analysis of RABV is commonly based on the N gene [4]. Previously, it was demonstrated that RABV genetic diversity has a strong geographic pattern throughout the world, which possibly results from the recent virus spread [5, 6]. Based on data received, all currently known RABV genetic variants can be divided globally into seven major groups [6]. Within these major groups, smaller genetic groups could be distinguished; thus, within the Cosmopolitan, and the Arctic/Arctic-like major groups, circulating in the Russian Federation six smaller groups were described in Russia: Arctic rabies (northern parts of Siberia), Arctic-like rabies (Khabarovsk Krai, Transbaikal region), Steppe rabies (Eurasian Steppe), Central European Russian rabies, Northeast European Rabies, and Caucasian rabies [6–8].

4. Rabies distribution

Currently, RABV is distributed globally and rabies infection is registered on all continents except Antarctica and, possibly, Australia. According to CDC data (https://www.cdc.gov/rabies/), the most (more than 90%) of all animal cases of rabies reported occur in wild animals; before 1960, most were in domestic animals. According to current data, the principal rabies hosts are wild carnivores and bats. Despite significant progress in the prevention and prophylaxis of rabies worldwide [9], rabies remains an important public health concern, especially in developing countries within Africa and Asia where rabies virus causes approximately 50,000 lethal cases per year [10]. Also, the official statistical data could be greatly underestimated due to the lack of systematic surveillance in some countries.

5. Rabies pathogenesis, prevention, and prophylaxis

Delivered into a wound through the bite or wound contamination with virus-containing biological liquids, the virus can replicate at the inoculation site [11].

After that, RABV reaches the sensory or motor neurons and then propagates up to the central nervous system by following neuronal connections. Such pathways through nervous tissue shield the virus from the host immune system, resulting in absence of early antibody response [12]. Being delivered to the central nervous system, the virus disseminates rapidly, and nearly all regions of the central nervous system may be affected. Nevertheless, the duration of the asymptomatic incubation period can be long-standing (two months on average), while the symptomatic period with clinical signs is rapid and severe (about one week).

Although rabies has the highest case fatality rate (100%), fortunately, it is a preventable disease. Postexposure prophylaxis consisting of rabies immune globulin or/and rabies vaccine is very effective in preventing the disease development when administered promptly after virus exposure has occurred. Also, very important measures to reduce the risk of RABV transmission to humans are vaccination of domestic animals against rabies and stray animal control programs.

Author details

Sergey Tkachev[1,2]

1 Institute of Fundamental Medicine and Biology, Kazan Federal University, Kazan, Russia

2 Institute of Chemical Biology and Fundamental Medicine SB RAS, Novosibirsk, Russia

*Address all correspondence to: sergey.e.tkachev@gmail.com

IntechOpen

References

[1] Knipe DM, Howley PM, editors.
Fields Virology. 6th ed. Philadelphia,
USA: Lippincott Williams & Wilkins,
a Wolters Kluwer Business; 2013

[2] Chenik M, Chebli K, Blondel D.
Translation initiation at alternate
in-frame AUG codons in the rabies virus
phosphoprotein mRNA is mediated by a
ribosomal leaky scanning mechanism.
Journal of Virology. 1995;**69**(2):707-712.
DOI: 10.1128/JVI.69.2.707-712.1995

[3] Kuzmin IV, Wu X, Tordo N,
Rupprecht CE. Complete genomes of
Aravan, Khujand, Irkut and West
Caucasian bat viruses, with special
attention to the polymerase gene and
non-coding regions. Virus Research.
2008;**136**(1-2):81-90. DOI: 10.1016/j.
virusres.2008.04.021

[4] Saito M, Oshitani H, Orbina JRC,
Tohma K, de Guzman AS, Kamigaki T,
et al. Genetic diversity and geographic
distribution of genetically distinct
rabies viruses in the Philippines.
PLoS Neglected Tropical Diseases.
2013;**7**:e2144. DOI: 10.1371/journal.
pntd.0002144

[5] Bourhy H, Reynes J-M, Dunham EJ,
Dacheux L, Larrous F, Huong VTQ,
et al. The origin and phylogeography
of dog rabies virus. The Journal of
General Virology. 2008;**89**:2673-2681.
DOI: 10.1099/vir.0.2008/003913-0

[6] Deviatkin AA, Lukashev AN,
Poleshchuk EM, Dedkov VG,
Tkachev SE, Sidorov GN, et al. The
phylodynamics of the rabies virus in
the Russian Federation. PLoS One.
2017;**12**(2):e0171855. DOI: 10.1371/
journal.pone.0171855

[7] Kuzmin IV, Botvinkin AD,
McElhinney LM, Smith JS, Orciari LA,
Hughes GJ, et al. Molecular
epidemiology of terrestrial rabies in the
former Soviet Union. Journal of

Wildlife Diseases. 2004;**40**:617-631.
DOI: 10.7589/0090-3558-40.4.617

[8] Metlin A, Rybakov S, Gruzdev K,
Neuvonen E, Huovilainen A. Genetic
heterogeneity of Russian, Estonian and
Finnish field rabies viruses. Archives of
Virology. 2007;**152**:1645-1654.
DOI: 10.1007/s00705-007-1001-6

[9] Dietzschold B, Faber M, Schnell MJ.
New approaches to the prevention and
eradication of rabies. Expert Review of
Vaccines. 2003;**2**:399-406. DOI: 10.1586/
14760584.2.3.399

[10] Knobel DL, Cleaveland S,
Coleman PG, Fèvre EM, Meltzer MI,
Miranda M, et al. Re-evaluating the
burden of rabies in Africa and Asia.
Bulletin of the World Health
Organization. 2005;**83**:360-366

[11] Murphy FA, Bauer SP. Early street
rabies virus infection in striated muscle
and later progression to the central
nervous system. Intervirology.
1974;**3**(4):256-268. DOI: 10.1159/
000149762

[12] Johnson N, Cunningham AF,
Fooks AR. The immune response to
rabies virus infection and vaccination.
Vaccine. 2010;**28**(23):3896-3901.
DOI: 10.1016/j.vaccine.2010.03.039

Chapter 2

The Early Development of the Vaccinia–Rabies Recombinant Vaccine Raboral®

Richard Lathe and Marie Paule Kieny

Abstract

The recombinant vaccinia–rabies vaccine, now known as Raboral®, has been widely used in Europe and North America to control/eliminate rabies in the principal wildlife vectors, and thus prevent human transmission. The origins of this vaccine are sometimes forgotten, although the formulation has not changed substantially in almost four decades. This groundbreaking vaccine was assembled by a team at a very young (at that time) genetic engineering company, Transgène, in Strasbourg, France. The joint leaders of the rabies vaccine team reflect, 36 years later, on the trials and tribulations that went hand in hand with the construction of the vaccine.

Keywords: Alsace, glycoprotein, Pasteur, rabies, Raboral, vaccine, vaccinia virus, wildlife

1. Introduction

Rabies is a devastating disease that is inexorably fatal, unless – as Louis Pasteur demonstrated [1] – it is rapidly treated by immunization. Even so, the vaccination regimen that Pasteur recommended is punishing, and brought its own risks of hyperinflammation. In the mid-20th century rabies was widespread among wildlife (principally foxes in Europe and raccoons in North America), and even in developed countries the bite of an infected animal was a death warrant if not immediately and intensively treated.

With the advent of genetic engineering (GE) technologies in the 1980s, the renowned Institut Mérieux in Lyon, France – established in 1897 by Marcel Mérieux, one of Louis Pasteur's assistants – brought a new task to the newly established GE company Transgène in Strasbourg: make a rabies vaccine. This chore was handed down to ourselves, two young postdoctoral scientists in the company.

Transgène, founded by Pierre Chambon and Philippe Kourilsky in 1979/1980, although being allocated half a floor in Pierre Chambon's institute at the University of Strasbourg (**Figure 1**), was not quite ready: all available resources, at the very beginning, were allocated to setting up all the essential GE ingredients – oligonucleotide synthesis, DNA sequencing (done manually on thin polyacrylamide gels using radiophosphorus), basic sequence analysis, simple expression vectors in bacteria, yeast, and mammalian cells, even making our own restriction enzymes. Other GE companies were well ahead, and had cloned and expressed key molecules such as growth hormone, interferons, and hepatitis B surface antigen. We were both overoptimistic and underweight.

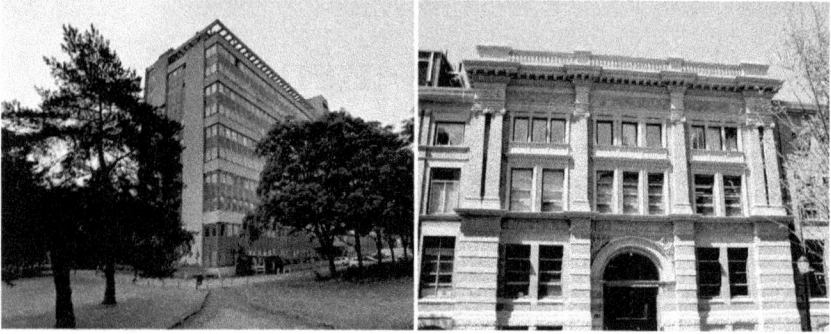

Figure 1.
Transgène and the Wistar Institute. (Left) The Laboratoire de Génétique Moléculaire des Eukaryotes (LGME) under Pierre Chambon at the Faculty of Medicine, University of Strasbourg (founded 1538), France, where Transgène was housed (6th floor) during the development of the rabies vaccine (1980s). The building was constructed in 1964 and was demolished in 2011 {https://www.archi-wiki.org/Adresse:Facult%C3%A9_de_m %C3%A9decine_(Strasbourg)}. (Right) Wistar Institute of Anatomy, Philadelphia, USA. The Wistar was founded in 1892, and the Wistar Institute Building was opened in 1894. Image courtesy Jeffrey M. Vinocur 2006. Images are reproduced under Wikipedia Creative Commons Attribution-ShareAlike License.

2. Construction of the Vaccine

But we set to. The Scientific Director of Transgène, Jean-Pierre Lecocq, established a collaboration with researchers at the Wistar Institute (**Figure 1**) under Hilary Koprowski (Philadelphia) who had obtained, for the first time, a cDNA copy of rabies virus glycoprotein at the end of 1981 [2, 3] – the key antigenic determinant of this virus. Beginning in early 1982, we expressed the cDNA in *E. coli*, *B. subtilis*, yeast, mammalian cells (reviewed in [4]). The pressure was on, we worked 7 days a week, so did our key technical staff; we were fuelled by Martha Argerich interpreting J.S. Bach on the tape player until long after the sun set over the Vosges hills (**Box 1**). The extracts were sent to the rabies expert in Philadelphia, Tadeusz Wiktor. He systematically vaccinated lab animals (mostly mice and hamsters) with the extracts, and then challenged them with street rabies virus. None survived.

We were dismayed, and ready to give up. Two developments changed everything. First, at a chance meeting with Peter Curtis (Wistar) he advised that there was a possible problem with his cDNA sequence – there appeared to be a mutation. Second, we were impressed by the growing achievements of recombinant vaccinia virus (the basis of the smallpox vaccine), inspired by Enzo Paoletti in 1983 [5], in eliciting immunity beyond what could be obtained with bacteria, yeasts, or even mammalian cells.

The mutation in the rabies glycoprotein cDNA was indeed suspect – a Pro to Leu mutation near the beginning of the mature protein sequence at a position that (to our minds) seemed to resemble known mutations at the beginning of the

It is singularly appropriate that the recombinant rabies vaccine should have been developed in Strasbourg, the central town of the province of Alsace, France. Louis Pasteur, famed for the first rabies vaccine, was born in the Jura hills (the southern extension of the Vosges – the hills of Alsace) and was Professor of Chemistry at Strasbourg University (formerly known as the Université Louis Pasteur) from 1849 to 1854, where he married Marie (also known as Louise) Laurent (the daughter of the Rector of the University), who for many years acted as his scientific assistant. The first patient to be treated against rabies, Joseph Meister (9 years old), traveled from Alsace to Pasteur's laboratory (then in Paris) for treatment [1]. The first fox to be inoculated with the new recombinant vaccine was in Malzéville, over the Vosges hills just 100 km from Strasbourg.

Box 1.
Rabies, Pasteur, and Alsace.

oncoprotein RAS (Gly to Asp, or Gly to Val) that entirely transform the structure and activity of the protein. The first thing we did was to correct the mutation. Something we had never done before, and this took months. In the key *Nature* paper

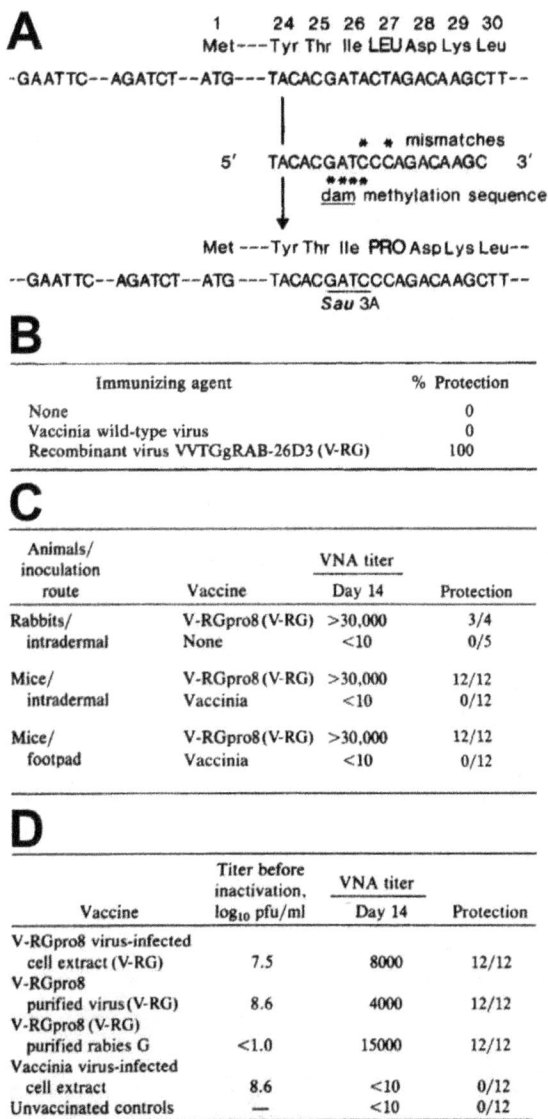

A

```
                        1        24 25 26 27 28 29 30
                        Met---Tyr Thr Ile LEU Asp Lys Leu

 -GAATTC--AGATCT--ATG---TACACGATACTAGACAAGCTT--

                                      *  *  mismatches
                     5'   TACACGATCCCAGACAAGC   3'
                              ****
                              dam methylation sequence

                        Met ---Tyr Thr Ile PRO Asp Lys Leu--

 --GAATTC--AGATCT--ATG --- TACACGATCCCAGACAAGCTT--
                               Sau 3A
```

B

Immunizing agent	% Protection
None	0
Vaccinia wild-type virus	0
Recombinant virus VVTGgRAB-26D3 (V-RG)	100

C

Animals/ inoculation route	Vaccine	VNA titer Day 14	Protection
Rabbits/ intradermal	V-RGpro8 (V-RG)	>30,000	3/4
	None	<10	0/5
Mice/ intradermal	V-RGpro8 (V-RG)	>30,000	12/12
	Vaccinia	<10	0/12
Mice/ footpad	V-RGpro8 (V-RG)	>30,000	12/12
	Vaccinia	<10	0/12

D

Vaccine	Titer before inactivation, $\log_{10}$ pfu/ml	VNA titer Day 14	Protection
V-RGpro8 virus-infected cell extract (V-RG)	7.5	8000	12/12
V-RGpro8 purified virus (V-RG)	8.6	4000	12/12
V-RGpro8 (V-RG) purified rabies G	<1.0	15000	12/12
Vaccinia virus-infected cell extract	8.6	<10	0/12
Unvaccinated controls	—	<10	0/12

Figure 2.
Construction and Activity of the Vaccinia-Based Recombinant Rabies Virus Raboral® VR-G. The recombinant was variously known as VR-G, VVTGgRAB-26D3, and VR-Gpro8. (A) Correction of a mutation in the N-terminus of the rabies glycoprotein coding sequence. Panel adapted, with permission, from [6]. (B) Protection from rabies using the live recombinant vaccine [6]. Mice were inoculated (intradermal) with 5 × 10⁵ PFU of VR-G or wild-type vaccinia, and challenged on day 15 by intracerebral inoculation of CDC culture-adapted street rabies virus (2400 LD50 units). All vaccinated animals survived. Panel adapted, with permission, from [6]. (C). Protection of rabbits and mice: inoculation was with 2 × 10⁸ PFU (intradermal) or 5 × 10⁷ (footpad) of VR-G; intracerebral challenge at day 14 was with 2400 (mice) or 24 000 (rabbits) mouse LD50 units of MD5951 street rabies virus. Panel adapted, with permission, from [7]. (D) Protection using inactivated VR-G. Vaccines were inactivated with β-propionolactone before intraperitoneal administration into mice. Challenge at day 14 was with 240 LD50 units of MD5951. Panel adapted, with permission, from [7].

the reader will see that, because our techniques were challenged, we took advantage of an artificial site for Dam methylase (that governs mismatch repair in *E. coli*) site to tip the balance in our favor (unheard of today) (**Figure 2A**). But it worked! We wonder how many rabies glycoprotein sequences circulating in the GE world today bear that same signature alteration.

The second thing we did was to get vaccinia up and running as a vehicle. We got into collaboration with Robert Drillien and Danièle Spehner at the Institut de Virologie on the same campus, and they supplied us with a microgram of vaccinia virus DNA. The key thymidine kinase gene – required for recombinational exchange with the vaccinia genome – had already been cloned by Robert, but we lacked a promoter to drive expression. We wanted the 7.5 K gene promoter, that had been worked up by researchers in the USA, but starting with only 1 microgram of DNA (the vaccinia genome is ~190 kb in length), given the state of the technology, cloning was near to impossible. In the event we turned to calculations of insert size, vector size, and absolute concentrations based on the physicochemistry of ligation [8, 9], and brewed up an optimum ligase mix. Only four clones were obtained. Two were 7.5 K in one orientation, and two were the same promoter in the other orientation! Were we lucky? No, in retrospect we would have got nothing had we not used the mathematics of the ligation reaction to get what we needed.

From there it moved quite rapidly. Ligate the promoter to the modified rabies G coding sequence, insert the construct into the vaccinia TK gene on a plasmid – then transfect the recombinant (TK-negative) plasmid into vaccinia virus-infected cells, and select chemically using bromodeoxyuridine (that kills TK-positive viruses). And we had our first vaccinia–rabies recombinant ('26D3').

This sped off to Tad Wiktor in Philadelphia. We waited what seems like an eternity, but he reported quickly back with his preliminary results: 'this is the best rabies vaccine I have ever seen' – it protected mice against severe rabies challenge (**Figure 2B–D**) better than any other rabies vaccine. And so it turned out – first published in September 1984 ([6, 7]; reviewed in [10–12]).

What lessons can be drawn, if any? Our first thought is that we worked as a team, there was no academic infighting, no bickering about authorships that is too common today, and we all worked day and night to see the project through. Even technical staff were there late in the evening and at weekends. Second, collaboration is essential: we could not have done this project without the participation of scientists both near (Robert Drillien and Danièle Spehner) and far {Tadeusz Wiktor (**Figure 3A**),

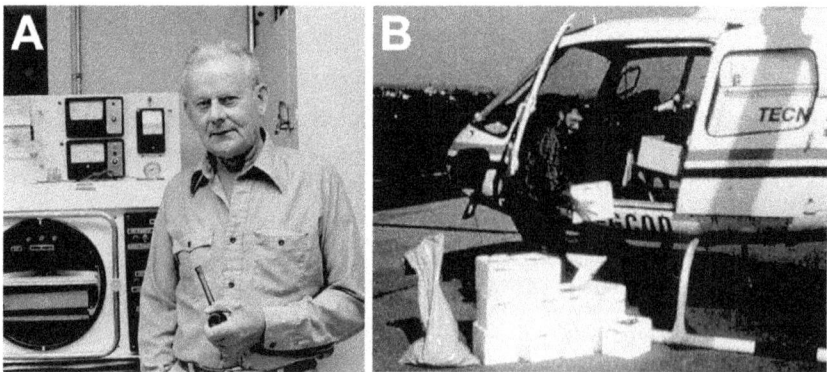

Figure 3.
Pioneering Rabies Vaccination. (A) Tadeusz J. Wiktor (1920–1985), rabies expert, Wistar Institute, who first tested the recombinant for efficacy. Photo courtesy of the Wistar Institute. (B) Loading vaccine baits into a helicopter during the first wildlife vaccination campaigns (Belgium, ca 1988; image collection M.P.K.).

Peter Curtis, and Hilary Koprowski}. Third, we wonder whether Martha Argerich and J.S. Bach played a role. In this day of P values, we would need to run the entire project again with a different musical background.

3. Vaccination of Wildlife

The vaccine was originally envisaged for human use, and steps were taken in this direction in collaboration with the Institut Mérieux. However, there was reluctance

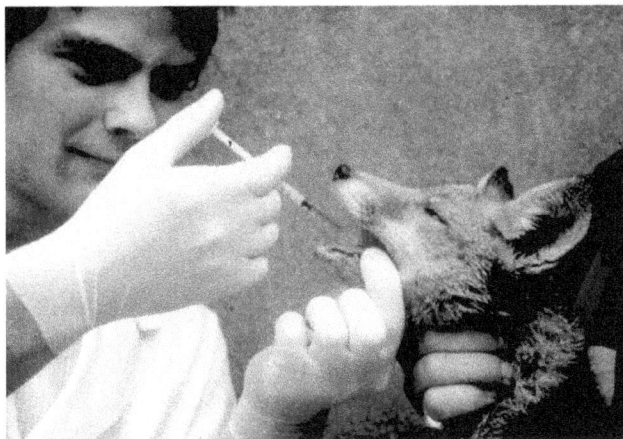

Figure 4.
Experimental vaccination of foxes, Malzéville, France, ca 1986 (image collection M.P.K.).

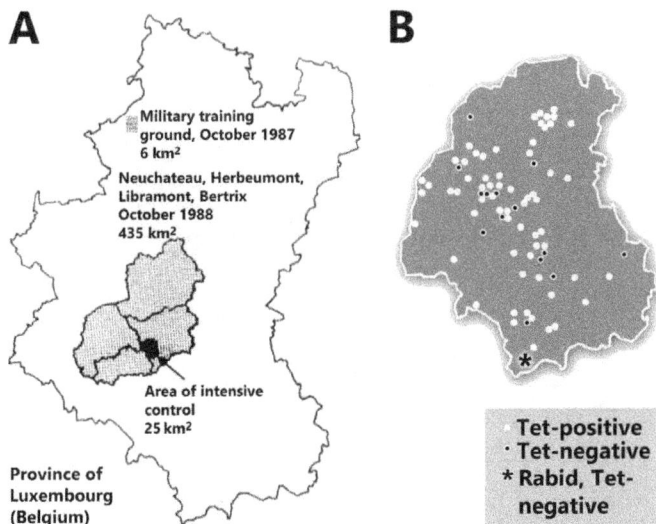

Figure 5.
First wildlife vaccination campaigns. Baits containing VRG were prepared from fish oil and protein. (A) Test areas in Belgium, 1987–1988. Vaccines were distributed at 15–50 baits per km²; uptake ranged from 27% at day 4 to 94% at day 223 (image collection M.P.K.). (B) Larger-scale field trial in a 2200 km² area of Belgium; distribution was at 15 baits per km²; the area was vaccinationed three times (1990–1991). Baits contained a tetracycline biomarker, and uptake determined from the presence of tetracycline (Tet; UV fluorescence in jaw) was 81% after the third phase. The single rabid fox detected after the campaign, at the periphery of the baited area, was Tet-negative. Image adapted, with permission, from [17].

to introduce a new vaccinia-based vaccine for human use because smallpox, the original target of vaccinia, had recently been declared eradicated by the World Health Organization (WHO) [13]. A committee of international experts including WHO representatives, who met in Bethesda, MD, in November 1984, did not envisage early human use [14]. However, because rabies is transmitted to humans principally from domestic dogs – that themselves acquire the infection from foxes (in Europe), and from raccoons and coyotes (in North America) – the next step was to try the new vaccine out for efficacy in animals. With support from Philippe Desmettre at the Institut Mérieux, Transgène was in touch with Pierre-Paul Pastoret in Belgium and colleagues at the French Ministry of Agriculture Rabies Research Station in Malzéville close to Nancy, and this was soon followed by the

Europe (including Russia)	
Austria	Eliminated (2006)
Belgium	Eliminated (1999)
Bulgaria	Reduction in seeded areas
Czech Republic	Eliminated (2002)
Estonia	Eliminated (2009)
France	Eliminated (1998)
Germany	Eliminated (2006)
Hungary	Reduction in seeded areas
Italy	Eliminated (1986/1995); then reduction
Latvia	Reduction in seeded areas
Lithuania	Reduction in seeded areas
Luxembourg	Eliminated (1999)
Poland	Reduction in seeded areas
Kaliningrad (Russia)	Reduction in seeded areas
Russia	Experimental
Slovakia	Eliminated (2006)
Slovenia	Reduction
Switzerland	Eliminated (1996)
Ukraine	Reduction
North America	
Canada	Reduction in seeded areas
United States	Reduction in seeded areas
Middle and Far East	
Israel	Reduction in seeded areas
Tunisia	Experimental
India	Experimental
China	Experimental

In many cases Raboral® was used in conjunction with conventional attenuated viruses, although Raboral® is the only vaccine licensed for use in the USA (http://www.raboral.com/about-rabies/raboral-v-rg). Data: key reviews are by Freuling et al. [18] and Maki et al. [19].

Table 1.
Wildlife Vaccination Campaigns Using Raboral®.

demonstration that oral administration of the vaccine (10^8 pfu) to foxes (**Figure 4**) gave complete protection against lethal challenge, and almost complete protection following administration in home-made bait [15], quickly followed by oral protection of raccoons in the USA by colleagues at the Wistar Institute [16].

This was expanded to small-trials followed by large-scale campaigns to eradicate sylvatic rabies in Europe and North America by dropping baits (e.g., chicken heads or artificial baits) seeded with live recombinant virus from helicopters (**Figure 3B**) according to a carefully planned routine (taking in mind the number of wildlife species per square kilometer, and the transmission factor R – what percentage of animals do we need to vaccinate to block propagation? – of current interest given the COVID pandemic). It worked. The first trials (**Figure 5**) demonstrated wide uptake by foxes and downturn of rabies cases. Using this vaccine, rabies has now been widely eliminated in many European countries; substantial reductions in rates of rabies in wildlife have been achieved in several areas of Eastern USA and Canada (**Table 1**) where active vaccination campaigns are ongoing (http://www.raboral. com/about-rabies/raboral-v-rg). Over 250 million doses of Raboral® have been distributed worldwide [19]. Although highly successful in Europe [18], campaigns in the USA and Canada are constrained because of rabies re-emergence through long-distance movements of carrier species such as arctic foxes [19].

4. Vaccinia-based vaccines for human use

The vaccina–rabies recombinant has never been approved for human use, even though vaccinia virus has been used widely across the world in our populations to eradicate smallpox, and the vaccinia–rabies recombinant is very much attenuated compared to standard strains of vaccinia. Notwithstanding, intense efforts have been made to develop vaccinia as an anticancer agent for direct prophylactic or curative use in human [20–23], but for recombinants expressing viral antigens few clinical trials have been carried out (with some exceptions; e.g., [24]). Efforts in the 1990s were invested into the development of viral vectors based on vaccinia derivatives such as modified virus Ankara (MVA) [25], or fowlpox or canarypox [26]. More recently., high levels of protective antibodies have been obtained against SARS coronavirus using vaccinia recombinants in experimental animals (e.g., [27–29]), and, given the threat of COVID-19, MVA-based recombinants are being actively explored in California [30] and Germany (https://www.vfa.de/de/englische-inhalte/vaccines-to-protect-against-covid-19) as potential vaccines against SARS-COV-2, the etiologic agent of COVID-19.

One potential way to circumvent safety concerns may be to employ inactivated recombinant vaccinia virions that display viral antigens at their surface: very substantial levels of protection were observed with chemically inactivated recombinant vaccinia–rabies virus [7], and this might afford an entry route for new human vaccines based on vaccinia – perhaps even at some stage including Raboral® or further attenuated derivatives, given that rabies in human remains a major concern in several regions such as India [31].

Acknowledgements

We acknowledge with appreciation the pivotal contributions of all our colleagues who made this work possible, notably Peter Curtis, Bill Wunner, Algis Anilionis, and Hilary Koprowski who provided the first rabies glycoprotein cDNA, Robert Drillien and Danièle Spehner for key help with vaccinia, Doris Schmitt and Karin Dott for superb technical assistance, all the teams at Transgène who helped with DNA sequencing, oligonucleotide synthesis, microbial gene expression systems, Tadeusz Wiktor for performing all the *in vivo* rabies challenge studies in Philadelphia, Pierre-Paul Pastoret in Belgium and Philippe Desmettre in France (and Charles Rupprecht and many others at the Wistar Institute) for enthusiastically speeding the transition to wildlife, the Institut Mérieux for sponsoring this work, and Jean-Pierre Lecocq, Philippe Kourilsky, and Pierre Chambon for supporting the project since inception.

Disclaimer

The views expressed herein are solely those of the authors and do not reflect the views of the WHO, Transgène SA, the INSERM, or of any other institution with which the authors are or have been associated.

Author details

Richard Lathe[1*] and Marie Paule Kieny[2*]

1 Division of Infection Medicine, University of Edinburgh Medical School, Edinburgh, UK

2 Institut National de la Santé et de la Recherche Médicale (INSERM), Paris, France

*Address all correspondence to: richard.lathe@ed.ac.uk
and marie-paule.kieny@inserm.fr

IntechOpen

References

[1] Nicolle J (1961) Louis Pasteur: A Master of Scientific Enquiry. Hutchinson, London.

[2] Anilionis A, Wunner WH, Curtis PJ (1981) Structure of the glycoprotein gene in rabies virus. Nature 294:275-278.

[3] Anilionis A, Wunner WH, Curtis PJ (1982) Amino acid sequence of the rabies virus glycoprotein deduced from its cloned gene. Comp Immunol Microbiol Infect Dis 5:27-32.

[4] Lecocq JP, Kieny MP, Lemoine Y, Drillien R, Wiktor T, Koprowski H, Lathe R (1985) New rabies vaccines: recombinant DNA approaches. In: Koprowski H, Plotkin SA (eds) World's Debt to Pasteur. Alan R. Liss, New York, pp. 259-271.

[5] Panicali D, Davis SW, Weinberg RL, Paoletti E (1983) Construction of live vaccines by using genetically engineered poxviruses: biological activity of recombinant vaccinia virus expressing influenza virus hemagglutinin. Proc Natl Acad Sci U S A 80:5364-5368.

[6] Kieny MP, Lathe R, Drillien R, Spehner D, Skory S, Schmitt D, Wiktor T, Koprowski H, Lecocq JP (1984) Expression of rabies virus glycoprotein from a recombinant vaccinia virus. Nature 312:163-166.

[7] Wiktor TJ, MacFarlan RI, Reagan KJ, Dietzschold B, Curtis PJ, Wunner WH, Kieny MP, Lathe R, Lecocq JP, Mackett M, et al. (1984) Protection from rabies by a vaccinia virus recombinant containing the rabies virus glycoprotein gene. Proc Natl Acad Sci U S A 81:7194-7198.

[8] Dugaiczyk A, Boyer HW, Goodman HM (1975) Ligation of EcoRI endonuclease-generated DNA fragments into linear and circular structures. J Mol Biol 96:171-184.

[9] Shore D, Langowski J, Baldwin RL (1981) DNA flexibility studied by covalent closure of short fragments into circles. Proc Natl Acad Sci U S A 78: 4833-4837.

[10] Lathe R, Kieny MP, Lecocq JP, Drillien R, Wiktor T, Koprowski H (1985) Immunization against rabies using a vaccinia-rabies recombinant virus expressing the surface glycoprotein. In: Lerner RA, Chanock RM, Brown F (eds) Vaccines 85. Cold Spring Harbor Laboratory, New York, pp. 157-162.

[11] Kieny MP, Desmettre P, Soulebot JP, Lathe R (1987) Rabies vaccine: traditional and novel approaches. Prog Vet Microbiol Immunol 3:73-111.

[12] Wiktor TJ, Kieny MP, Lathe R (1988) New generation of rabies vaccine: vaccinia-rabies glycoprotein recombinant virus. In: Kurstak E, Marusyk RG, Murphy FA, Van Regenmortel MHV (eds) Applied Virology Research. Plenum Press, New York, pp. 69-90.

[13] Fenner F, Henderson DA, Arita I, Jezek Z, Ladnyi ID (1988) Smallpox and Its Eradication. World Health Organization, Geneva.

[14] Ada GL, Brown F, et al. (1985) Recombinant vaccinia viruses as live virus vectors for vaccine antigens: memorandum from a WHO/USPHS/NIBSC meeting. Bull World Health Organ 63:471-477.

[15] Blancou J, Kieny MP, Lathe R, Lecocq JP, Pastoret PP, Soulebot JP, Desmettre P (1986) Oral vaccination of the fox against rabies using a live recombinant vaccinia virus. Nature 322:373-375.

[16] Rupprecht CE, Wiktor TJ, Johnston DH, Hamir AN, Dietzschold B, Wunner WH, Glickman LT, Koprowski H (1986) Oral immunization and

protection of raccoons (Procyon lotor) with a vaccinia-rabies glycoprotein recombinant virus vaccine. Proc Natl Acad Sci U S A 83:7947-7950.

[17] Brochier B, Kieny MP, Costy F, Coppens P, Bauduin B, Lecocq JP, Languet B, Chappuis G, Desmettre P, Afiademanyoll K, Libois R, Pastoret P-P (1991) Large-scale eradication of rabies using recombinant vaccinia–rabies vaccine. Nature 354:520-522.

[18] Freuling CM, Hampson K, Selhorst T, Schröder R, Meslin FX, Mettenleiter TC, Müller T (2013) The elimination of fox rabies from Europe: determinants of success and lessons for the future. Philos Trans R Soc Lond B Biol Sci 368:20120142.

[19] Maki J, Guiot AL, Aubert M, Brochier B, Cliquet F, Hanlon CA, King R, Oertli EH, Rupprecht CE, Schumacher C, Slate D, Yakobson B, Wohlers A, Lankau EW (2017) Oral vaccination of wildlife using a vaccinia-rabies-glycoprotein recombinant virus vaccine (RABORAL V-RG®): a global review. Vet Res 48:57.

[20] Lathe R, Kieny MP, Gerlinger P, Clertant P, Guizani I, Cuzin F, Chambon P (1987) Tumour prevention and rejection with recombinant vaccinia. Nature 326:878-880.

[21] Hareuveni M, Gautier C, Kieny MP, Wreschner D, Chambon P, Lathe R (1990) Vaccination against tumor cells expressing breast cancer epithelial tumor antigen. Proc Natl Acad Sci U S A 87:9498-9502.

[22] Meneguzzi G, Cerni C, Kieny MP, Lathe R (1991) Immunization against human papillomavirus type 16 tumor cells with recombinant vaccinia viruses expressing E6 and E7. Virology 181:62-69.

[23] Quoix E, Lena H, Losonczy G, Forget F, Chouaid C, Papai Z, Gervais R, Ottensmeier C, Szczesna A, Kazarnowicz A, Beck JT, Westeel V, Felip E, Debieuvre D, Madroszyk A, Adam J, Lacoste G, Tavernaro A, Bastien B, Halluard C, Palanché T, Limacher JM (2016) TG4010 immunotherapy and first-line chemotherapy for advanced non-small-cell lung cancer (TIME): results from the phase 2b part of a randomised, double-blind, placebo-controlled, phase 2b/3 trial. Lancet Oncol 17:212-223.

[24] Pitisuttithum P, Rerks-Ngarm S, Bussaratid V, Dhitavat J, Maekanantawat W, Pungpak S, Suntharasamai P, Vanijanonta S, Nitayapan S, Kaewkungwal J, Benenson M, Morgan P, O'Connell RJ, Berenberg J, Gurunathan S, Francis DP, Paris R, Chiu J, Stablein D, Michael NL, Excler JL, Robb ML, Kim JH (2011) Safety and reactogenicity of canarypox ALVAC-HIV (vCP1521) and HIV-1 gp120 AIDSVAX B/E vaccination in an efficacy trial in Thailand. PLoS One 6:e27837.

[25] Mayr A (1999) Historical review of smallpox, the eradication of smallpox and the attenuated smallpox MVA vaccine (article in German). Berl Munch Tierarztl Wochenschr 112:322-328.

[26] Taylor J, Tartaglia J, Rivière M, Duret C, Languet B, Chappuis G, Paoletti E (1994) Applications of canarypox (ALVAC) vectors in human and veterinary vaccination. Dev Biol Stand 82:131-135.

[27] Bisht H, Roberts A, Vogel L, Bukreyev A, Collins PL, Murphy BR, Subbarao K, Moss B (2004) Severe acute respiratory syndrome coronavirus spike protein expressed by attenuated vaccinia virus protectively immunizes mice. Proc Natl Acad Sci U S A 101:6641-6646.

[28] Chen Z, Zhang L, Qin C, Ba L, Yi CE, Zhang F, Wei Q, He T, Yu W, Yu J, Gao H, Tu X, Gettie A, Farzan M, Yuen KY, Ho DD (2005) Recombinant modified vaccinia virus Ankara expressing the spike glycoprotein of

severe acute respiratory syndrome coronavirus induces protective neutralizing antibodies primarily targeting the receptor binding region. J Virol 79:2678-2688.

[29] Ishii K, Hasegawa H, Nagata N, Mizutani T, Morikawa S, Suzuki T, Taguchi F, Tashiro M, Takemori T, Miyamura T, Tsunetsugu-Yokota Y (2006) Induction of protective immunity against severe acute respiratory syndrome coronavirus (SARS-CoV) infection using highly attenuated recombinant vaccinia virus DIs. Virology 351:368-380.

[30] Chiuppesi F, Salazar MD, Contreras H, Nguyen VH, Martinez J, Park Y, Nguyen J, Kha M, Iniguez A, Zhou Q, Kaltcheva T, Levytskyy R, Ebelt ND, Kang TH, Wu X, Rogers TF, Manuel ER, Shostak Y, Diamond DJ, Wussow F (2020) Development of a multi-antigenic SARS-CoV-2 vaccine candidate using a synthetic poxvirus platform. Nat Commun 11:6121.

[31] Chatterjee P (2009) India's ongoing war against rabies. Bull World Health Organ 87:890-891.

Chapter 3

The Diagnosis, Clinical Course, Treatment, and Prevention of the Rabies Virus

Jaida Hopkins, Samantha Sweck and Sean Richards

Abstract

Rabies, despite available vaccines, causes approximately 55,000 deaths every year. Diagnosing relies on noting physical behaviors such as hydrophobia, vomiting, fever, behavior changes, paralysis, and consciousness, as well as, using several methodologies to molecularly detect the presence of the virus. RABV often enters through a bite wound given that it is transmissible through saliva. Infection spreads from muscle fibers into the peripheral nervous system traveling to the central nervous system. Infection of the central nervous system can lead to encephalitis (furious rabies) or acute flaccid paralysis (paralytic rabies). Treatment relies heavily on the time of exposure. If the patient is diagnosed prior to being symptomatic, post-exposure prophylaxis (PEP) can be administered. However, once the patient has begun displaying symptoms, therapy success rates sharply decline. Prevention includes vaccinating during both pre- and post-exposures, as well as utilizing Stepwise Approach towards Rabies Elimination (SARE) to aid impoverished countries in declining their rabies mortality rates.

Keywords: rabies virus, RABV, diagnosis, treatment, prevention

1. Introduction

Rabies, an RNA virus from the genus Lyssavirus, also known as RABV, is a lethal pathogen to several species [1]. The evolutionary history of the virus suggests that its most recent ancestor likely diverged into two descendants, one infecting bats, the other infecting dogs. Once domesticated dogs became infected in the Old World, humans became the next target. Evolutionary biology tells us that rabies likely did not exist in the New World prior to the settlement of Europeans but was common throughout Europe, Asia, and Africa well before the discovery of the Americas [2].

RABV is transmitted through the saliva of an infected individual into the bloodstream of a healthy individual, typically via a bite, but possible through other wounds or ocular route. Upon infection, there are two ways the virus may manifest: furious and paralytic. Furious rabies often presents itself with bouts of anxiety, irritability, phobias, and many other symptoms that will later be discussed. Paralytic rabies has some common symptoms with furious rabies, however, paralysis is the most notable symptom just prior to death [3].

According to the CDC in 2015, nearly 60,000 human deaths occurred on average each year. Statistically, this can be interpreted as 1 human death every nine minutes [4]. Despite its large impact globally, the virus is relatively diminutive. The rabies virus has evolutionarily reduced its single-stranded RNA genome to only five genes. These genes encode five proteins, three of which make up the ribonucleoprotein (RNP) complex; the other two form the virus's envelope [5].

While the rabies virus has been heavily researched, lives continue to be lost. There is a great understanding of the epidemiology of the virus, however little is understood about the pathogenesis. Herein, the findings regarding the diagnosis, clinical course, treatment, and prevention of the rabies virus are summarized as well as data gaps in research and understanding of this pathogen.

2. Diagnostics

Once the patient has become infected, the incubation period can be as short as 5 days or as long as 2 years. However, it is common for symptoms to occur 20–90 days after initial exposure [6]. Nevertheless, there are several techniques for diagnosing a patient during and after the incubation period.

2.1 Physical symptoms

As mentioned previously, the two ways the rabies virus may present itself is paralytic and furious symptoms. A patient with paralytic rabies will show progressive paralysis until death. If infection occurred due to a bite, the paralysis typically starts around the wounded area, spreading outwards. It is also common for patients to have a fever, vomiting, weakness in muscles, and myalgia prior to the paralysis [7].

Furious rabies often presents itself with more obvious symptoms. The infected individual commonly displays mood swings, unregulated consciousness, phobias, especially hydrophobia, as well as spasms of the respiratory system [1, 8]. Other symptoms may include a cough, psychosis, delirium, and difficulties swallowing [9].

2.2 Neuroimaging

For both furious and paralytic rabies, magnetic resonance imaging (MRI) will produce the same key diagnostic images. When symptoms first arise in the prodromal phase, progression in hypersignal T2 changes can be seen around the brachial plexus and the spinal nerve roots associated with the extremity of infection origin. The main MRI feature is increased T2 signal (seen on T2 and FLAIR sequences) in the affected parts of the brain and spinal cord, with a predilection for grey matter structures including basal ganglia, thalami, hypothalami, limbic system, and brainstem. The abnormal hypersignal T2 changes will continue to progress as the patient enters a coma. Once in the comatose phase, the contrast will enhance around the spinal cord, nerve roots located at the sine and cranial region, deep grey matter, brain stem, limbic structures, and thalamus (**Figure 1**) [8].

Another study noted that lesions could be seen throughout different areas of the neuroaxis. They, too, found that paralytic and furious rabies present the same MRI indications, however, they are more noticeable in the paralytic form. The blood–brain barrier often shows no sign of damage until the patient reaches the comatose state. Imaging of the blood–brain barrier has greatly improved as new techniques such as diffusion-weighted and diffusion tensor imaging can capture objective and subjective data [11].

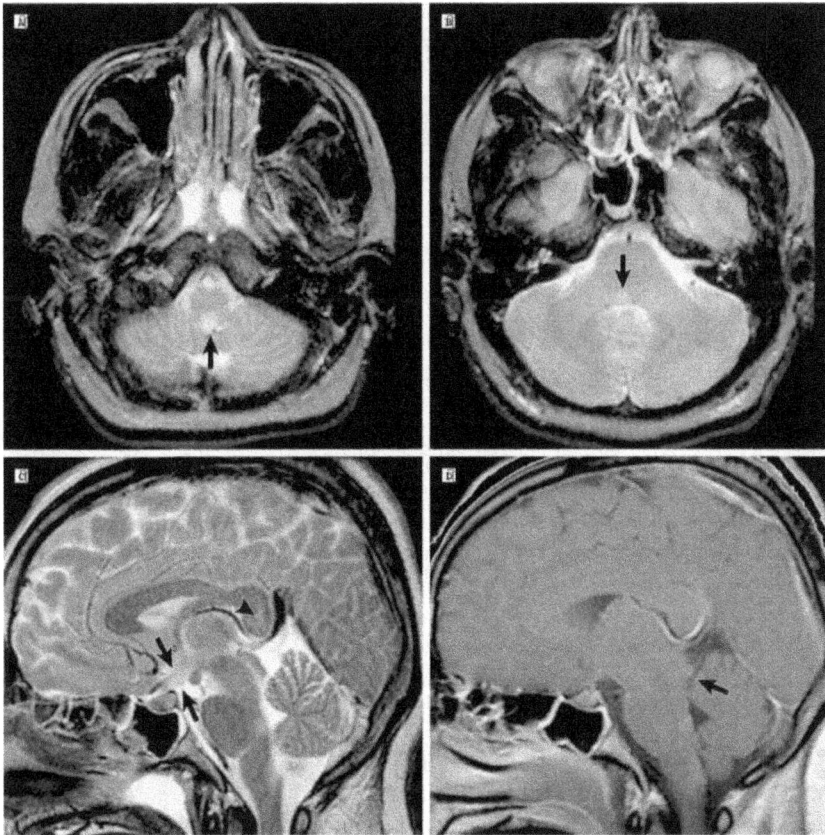

Figure 1.
Magnetic resonance images with arrows pointing to high focal areas (A. dorsal medulla, B. pons, C. hypothalamus, and D. splenium of corpus callosum) of an infected patient with furious rabies [10].

2.3 Testing techniques

There are several techniques used to diagnose a patient with a rabies infection; including reverse transcription polymerase chain reaction (rtPCR) analysis, fluorescent antibody test (FAT), tissue culturing, and viral antibody neutralization [12, 13]. The FAT assay has long been a microbiological standard for diagnosing rabies (and other viral infections). Fluorescent antibody virus neutralisation (FAVN) test is also used to diagnose rabies [13]. The CDC recommends a direct form of FAT to detect the rabies virus in animals ante-mortem, however, the animal is usually euthanized after detection and brain tissue samples taken to solidify the diagnosis post-mortem. However, diagnosis in humans requires several different types of methods such as direct rapid immunohistochemistry testing, the use of electron microscopy, and reverse transcriptase-polymerase chain reactions on biological samples (**Figure 2**) [15].

Another test utilizing immunohistochemistry, known as the direct rapid immunohistochemistry test (dRIT) is a specific form of histology because it employs antibodies unique to RABV. While this testing method can give a reliable result in less than an hour, retrieving brain samples is very invasive [16].

Samples can also be viewed using electron microscopy. When Negri bodies are located in samples, electron miscopy can give a clear depiction of the bullet-shaped

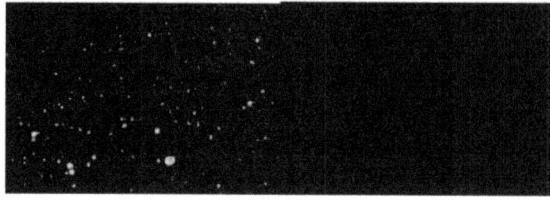

Figure 2.
These images show the comparison of a positive direct FAT result (left) and a negative direct FAT result (right) [14].

rabies virus being produced. A colloid can be used to compare the virus size to further interpret the image, however shape and size alone are not enough to identify with confidence [17].

Saliva and skin samples can be used for identifying the presence of RABV. rtPCR can be used to confirm or oppose the results of FAT test results. Because RABV is a single-stranded RNA virus, rtPCR can help transform RNA into DNA through amplification for analysis of a complement to a rabies-specific primer. This is often achieved by inoculating suckling mice and retrieving brain or kidney samples after death [15, 18].

2.4 Patients with psychiatric disorders

Given that the rabies virus significantly impacts the central nervous system, it is not uncommon for hallucinations, manic episodes, anxiety, and bouts of paranoia to be present in an infected patient [19, 20]. However, these are also common symptoms of psychiatric disorders such as schizophrenia. While it is rare, it is possible that correct RABV diagnosis may be complicated by a previous diagnosis of psychiatric disorders. Patients suffering from hypochondriasis could elicit psuedorabies [20]. In several case studies with reports of hypochondriasis, patients did not respond to therapies and often attempt suicide multiple times [20, 21]. While these situations are rare, they should be noted when diagnosing patients with certainty.

3. Clinical course

3.1 Pathophysiology

The most common entry point for RABV is through the bite of an infected individual as rabies resides in saliva [22]. However, transmission from organ transplants and aerosol droplets have also been recorded [23–25]. Upon entry, an incubation period often takes place in the myocytes, and rarely fibrocytes, where the virus attaches to the G-protein of the cells, enters through pinocytosis or fusion, and replicates in the cytoplasm of the cells [5, 24]. Virions will replicate with little to no immune response until the virus interacts with and infects a nerve cell. The rabies virus gains access to the nervous system by binding to the nicotinic acetylcholine receptors on the postsynaptic membrane at the neuromuscular junction [26]. From the point of nerve cell infection, the virus will travel via axon transport through the nervous system, eventually reaching the brainstem to give rise to either encephalitis or acute flaccid paralysis [7, 27]. The incubation periods are highly variable depending on the dosage of the virus. However, in humans, the incubation period is often >1–3 months. Canine incubation periods are most commonly less than 60 days [26, 28].

Once infection is recognized by the immune system, cytokine, IgM, and IgG antibody production increases [5]. Specific cytokines, Interleukin-1β (IL-1β) and TNFα, are thought to be the reason inflammation of the central nervous system occurs post-exposure [29]. The presence of these cytokines initiate a cascade reaction, upregulating proteins necessary for the inflammatory response such as the major histocompatibility complex and adhesion molecules. These proteins then interact with leukocytes to allow the blood brain barrier to become more permeable, thus causing an immune response leading to encephalitis [30]. As for the natural defense against rabies, RABV signals a series of molecular cascades that initiates type I interferon responses that have antiviral properties, decreasing the pathogenicity of rabies [31]. However, to artificially aid the natural response, there is heavy research on the potential to activate dendritic cells which subsequently enhance the activity of interleukin proteins and high mobility group box 1 (HMBG1) to enhance immunogenicity [32, 33].

4. Treatment

Although the rabies disease has been documented for thousands of years, it is still largely considered incurable after the onset of symptoms [34]. This is due to the small window of time during which aggressive treatment is practical and effective. With that knowledge, most often treatment resolves to be mostly palliative with aggressive treatment proving to be essentially ineffective after RABV is established in the patient.

4.1 Aggressive approach

If a patient presents for treatment early in the process of the clinical disease, the choice may be made to apply an aggressive approach. At this point, the patient must be immediately admitted to an intensive care hospital and post-exposure prophylaxis (PEP) should be administered [26]. PEP consists of immediate washing of the wound with soap and water, a post-exposure vaccination, and injection of an anti-rabies immunoglobulin (RIG) directly into the wound [35].

Active immunization has evolved greatly since the first rabies vaccine was developed and administered in 1885 [36, 37]. Louis Pasteur is credited with this first vaccine that consisted of injecting the patient with homogenates of RABV-infected rabbit spinal cord multiple times over a period of days. The initial injection was believed to be fully inactivated after an extended desiccation period, and each subsequent inoculation was increasingly more virulent as the desiccation period was decreased. While this was found to be somewhat effective, two major issues presented themselves. First, the inactivation of the RABV was inconsistent which led to some patients becoming infected after receiving the vaccine. Second, there was an inequity in the supply of the RABV-infected rabbits and the demand of the human population. These were rectified with the introduction of RABV-infected sheep and goat brain vaccines [36, 37]. These new vaccines were inactivated via chemical agents such as phenol; this proved to be much more consistent. However, soon it was understood that vaccines produced from mature brain material contained an excess of myelin which caused sensitization and ultimately killed the patients [38]. From this discovery emerged the current methodology by which rabies vaccines are created. Chick embryos served the same role as the previous tissues, but they have markedly less myelin due to the young age [39]. The same can be said of the lines of human diploid cells infected with fixed RABV for vaccines [36, 37]. In the United States, there are two CDC-approved vaccines: the human diploid cell culture vaccine (HDCV) and the purified chick embryo cell culture vaccine (PCECV) [15].

The post-exposure vaccine is primarily an intramuscular vaccine that ought to be given on day 0, 3, 7, 14, and 30 [36]. An intradermal vaccine has recently been developed in an attempt to decrease the amount of vaccine needed per injection [40]. While the decreased cost of the vaccine is an attractive option, intradermal injections are generally considered more difficult which could decrease the effectiveness of the vaccine due to improper injections. The World Health Organization (WHO) strongly recommends purified cell culture and embryonated egg-based vaccines [41].

Although the vaccines have been proven to stimulate an appropriate immune response to RABV, this immune response is often too delayed to prevent the virus from entering the nerves [42]. With this knowledge, passive immunization is recommended for all patients that have no previous history with the disease or a pre-exposure vaccination. At this time, two types of rabies immunoglobulin are available – human rabies immunoglobulin (HRIG) and equine rabies immunoglobulin (ERIG). These have been used since the 1970's to temporarily increase the concentration of rabies virus neutralizing antibodies (RVNA) specifically at the site of exposure [43]. If the patient has multiple bites or wounds, the RIG needs to be applied at each site to be effective [44]. HRIG is to be administered at a dosage or 20 IU/kg while the recommended dosage for ERIG is 40 IU/kg [42, 44]. Due to higher odds of sensitization as well as quicker elimination of the RVNA, HRIG is generally the most preferred option for passive immunization. However, it is approximately five times more expensive than ERIG. This results in a major deficiency in many of the countries most in need of rabies treatment [44].

Because the available RIGs are generally inaccessible to developing countries, WHO encouraged researchers to pursue synthetization of a human monoclonal antibodies (mAbs) cocktail that can be used to treat rabies [45]. At this time, there are a number of rabies mAbs products in clinical trials, but none have been approved by the US Food and Drug Administration [46]. In 2018, WHO officially adjusted their recommendations for treatment of rabies to include mAbs products in place of RIG if available [46].

A protocol known as the Milwaukee Protocol was presented as a potential cure in the late 20th century, but it has since been proven to be inconsistent and generally ineffective in reverting or curing the patient of the disease [47–49]. This protocol consisted of an induced coma and one or more antivirals. The coma was soon determined to be ineffective. It is now recommended that sedation should be limited to prevent the use of ventilatory support if possible [48, 49].

Antivirals could serve an important role in the treatment of the rabies virus as they act as inhibitors of viral replication. An effective antiviral could slow the progression of the rabies virus enough for the patient's innate immune response to develop and react appropriately. However, at this time, there are few antivirals supported for the treatment of RABV. Ribavirin is a purine analogue that acts as an RNA mutagen and has shown to be clinically effective for multiple viruses including Hepatitis C and Lassa fever virus [50, 51]. Despite its inclusion in the sporadically effective Milwaukee Protocol, it has repeatedly proven to be ineffective against the rabies virus. Interferon-α (IFN-α) is a signaling protein used to trigger an immune response which has been shown to limit RABV spreading in mice trials [50, 51]. However, additional trials in which primates were administered intramuscular and intrathecal IFN-α determined the effects of immediate inoculation to be incomplete while the effects of delayed inoculation were nonexistent [52, 53]. Six human patients have been treated with IFN-α on two different dosage schedules and despite evidence of increased IFN in serum and CSF, there was no evidence of a beneficial effect on the disease itself [54]. Another therapy previously included in the Milwaukee Protocol is ketamine [50, 51]. At low concentrations, approximately

1 µM, ketamine works as a non-competitive antagonist of the N-methyl-D-aspartate (NMDA) receptor which causes a state of dissociative anesthesia. A study from 1991 showed that a high concentration of ketamine could induce inhibitory effects on the RABV genome transcription [55]. Since that time, multiple other trials using neuron cultures and infected mice have produced evidence that ketamine is generally ineffective against the disease [56]. With that knowledge, it is believed that ketamine should not be used for treatment of the rabies virus until further studies produce more promising results. Amantadine is the third and final antiviral that was considered in the Milwaukee Protocol [47, 51]. It is a synthetic inhibitor of viral replication by impeding the release of viral genetic material into the host cell. Although amantadine demonstrated some interference in cellular trials, it failed in animal trials [57]. Minocycline, a broad spectrum antimicrobial, was considered for RABV treatment as it has proven benefits for multiple other viruses [58]. However, when applied to rabies-infected animals, Minocycline caused a number of harmful effects causing an increase in mortality [59].

More recently, researchers have addressed the use of favipiravir in treatment of rabies [50]. Available for influenza treatment in some countries, favipiravir has shown some activity against the rabies virus in mice trials [60]. Continued studies are needed to assess the future of this and other antivirals. It ought to be noted that despite variations in the effectiveness of these antivirals, all have shown that an early start of treatment greatly improves the efficacy of these therapies.

4.2 Palliative care

As previously mentioned, there is a small window of effectiveness for an aggressive treatment of RABV; after that window has passed, the focus of treatment is purely one of comfort for the patient. Many patients develop phobias that will likely require seclusion in a calm, quiet room. Although there is little to no evidence of human-to-human transmission, visitors and medical professionals need to be cautious of potential contamination via the patient's secretion [61]. Dehydration is a major concern as paralytic rabies often inhibits the patient's ability to swallow and furious rabies can cause intense hydrophobia. Treatment for the dehydration is typically a secured intravenous line. If additional nutrients are needed, they can be administered through the same line.

Rabies typically causes a generalized inflammation that induces a fever, but it can also trigger a neurogenic (central) fever as well [62]. Many antipyretics, such as acetaminophen and ibuprofen, have been successfully used to treat the generalized fever. However, those are generally ineffective towards the central fever. There is some evidence to support the use of baclofen, bromocriptine, chlorpromazine, and morphine in the treatment of a central fever [63]. However, these have not been studied specifically for a rabies-induced central fever and so practitioners should be mindful of potential side effects. Additionally, these drugs are rarely available in the developing countries where RABV is most prevalent [61]. In this case, external, physical means of cooling the patient can be used as needed.

The majority of patients infected with furious RABV develop intense agitation and fear. A variety of sedatives and tranquilizers are used to calm these symptoms. Because benzodiazepines are included on the WHO's list of essential medicines, they are commonly used to treat rabies-induced agitation as well as many other forms [61]. They can be administered intramuscularly, intravenously, or intrarectally as needed. However, as previously mentioned, it is important to administer any sedative slowly to ensure the patient retains consciousness and does not lose respiratory function [64].

Lastly, clinicians will likely need to address the patient's pain level. This can be accomplished using opioids such as morphine or other highly effective analgesics. These can be delivered intravenously, intramuscularly, intrarectally, or even transdermally as needed [61]. Although many of these methods of treatment are expensive and generally unlikely to cure a patient once rabies symptoms are present, palliative care is a responsibility of caretakers and clinicians.

5. Prevention

Due to the general ineffectiveness of post-exposure treatment, the rabies virus has a remarkably high mortality rate despite the availability of vaccines that have shown a near perfect success rate when administered prior to infection. This indicates that the main issue with prevention is the lack of accessibility in the impoverished countries of Asia and Africa. In 2015, the World Health Organization (WHO) and the World Organization for Animal Health (OIE) with the help of the Food and Agriculture Organization of the United Nations (FAO) set a goal to rid the world of dog-mediated rabies by 2030 (Zero by 30) [65]. After assessing cost and general accessibility, it was decided that the best way to eliminate dog-mediated rabies is to vaccinate dogs rather than humans. Vaccinating at least 70% of dogs should effectively break the cycle of rabies transmission.

To reach this goal, WHO, OIE, FAO and many smaller agencies collaborated to create the Stepwise Approach towards Rabies Elimination (SARE) [66, 67]. A similar stepwise approach proved successful in the elimination of fox RABV from Europe [68]. SARE consists of five stages for each country to work through. Stage 0 is simply the lack of information and data on RABV cases in a country where rabies is believed to be present. Stage 1 is an assessment phase in which data are gathered to determine the extent to which RABV pervades the country of interest. During this phase, the government assesses the current guidelines or structures in place as well as collects and analyzes all available data on previous or existing RABV cases. The beginning of an action plan is usually concocted in Stage 1. Evolution of this plan happens in Stage 2; it is important to develop an understanding of the available funding at this point as that has been the biggest limitation for developing countries in the past. Stage 3 is the implementation of the country's rabies control strategy. During this phase, the plan will likely need to be adapted to address any challenges that arise; these may include the exposure of wildlife reservoirs of RABV such as the fox rabies previously found in Europe. When reported human cases have decreased to zero, the country will shift into Stage 4 – elimination of dog RABV. This requires the maintenance of the reduced dog-to-human rabies transmission as well as continued implementation of the action plan to continue to reduce dog rabies cases. Lastly, in Stage 5, the country must develop a post-elimination strategy to maintain the freedom from human and dog rabies.

While the SARE tool has been developed to be adaptable enough to succeed worldwide, there are likely to be some setbacks in the different landscapes. Specifically, areas of poverty will be constrained by the financial resources they can acquire. Many parts of Asia have political instability that will greatly challenge the need for nation-wide commitment to this goal. Similarly, Africa's linguistic and cultural complexity will oppose the need for excellent communication and tracking [66]. Ultimately, it will take a dedicated and educated global population to eliminate rabies as a whole; until then, vaccinating animals and at-risk populations is the most efficient means of prevention.

6. Conclusion

This chapter served to outline the diagnosis, clinical course, treatment, and prevention of the RNA virus RABV. A swift rabies's diagnosis is imperative to ensure the patient's greatest chance of survival. Clinicians may utilize many techniques such as MRI, rtPCR, FAT, FAVN, dRIT, and electron microscopy to diagnose patients before physical symptoms arise. The same methods can be used to confirm a diagnosis after the patient presents with symptoms if needed. Rabies can present in patients in the furious or paralytic form. Although these cause very different physical symptoms, the pathophysiology is very similar. Generally initiated by a bite or other wound, the virus will incubate in the myocytes nearest the entry point and replicate undetected for an average of 1–3 months. Eventually, the virus will infect a nerve cell and travel through axon transport to the CNS at which point it will cause encephalitis or paralysis. Once the virus has infiltrated the CNS, it is essentially incurable. However, if detected early, patients can receive PEP - a combination of active and passive immunization most frequently in the form of a cell culture vaccine and a dose of RIG. At this time, there are no antivirals considered to be effective for treating RABV. If the virus becomes established in the patient, the treatment plan is adjusted to ensure the most comfort for the patient and their loved ones. This most often consists of a variety of sedatives, pain management, antipyretics, and fluids. Due to the great lethality of RABV in humans, multiple global organizations have banded together to attempt to eradicate the modern world of the rabies virus. The Zero by 30 movement strives to implement a stepwise method to eliminate dog-mediated rabies cases worldwide by 2030. This is believed to be possible if 70% or more of the dog population is vaccinated against rabies. In combination with the vaccination goal, Zero by 30 also encourages countries to implement educational standards on rabies, bite prevention, and responsible pet ownership.

At this time, the community of RABV researchers need to be working to improve current treatment options in order to decrease the number of RABV-related deaths. This might be done by developing a mAb alternative to the too-expensive RIG options or finding an effective antiviral either currently on the market or newly developed. The release of additional rabies vaccines for humans would also help to lower the price and improve the accessibility in a way that would benefit the highly affected countries.

Conflict of interest

The authors declare no conflict of interest.

Author details

Jaida Hopkins, Samantha Sweck and Sean Richards*
University of Tennessee, Chattanooga, USA

*Address all correspondence to: seanrichards.utc@gmail.com

IntechOpen

References

[1] Jackson AC. Human Rabies: a 2016 Update. Current Infectious Disease Reports. 2016;18(11):38.

[2] Velasco-Villa A, Mauldin MR, Shi M, Escobar LE, Gallardo-Romero NF, Damon I, et al. The history of rabies in the Western Hemisphere. Antiviral Research. 2017;146:221-232.

[3] Mitrabhakdi E, Shuangshoti S, Wannakrairot P, Lewis RA, Susuki K, Laothamatas J, et al. Difference in neuropathogenetic mechanisms in human furious and paralytic rabies. Journal of the Neurological Sciences. 2005;238(1):3-10.

[4] Every 9 Minutes, Someone in the World Dies of Rabies [press release]. Centers for Disease Control and Prevention2015.

[5] Rupprecht CE. Rhabdoviruses: Rabies Virus. 1996. In: Medical Microbiology [internet] [Internet]. Galveston (TX): University of Texas Medical Branch at Galveston. 4th. Available from: https://www.ncbi.nlm.nih.gov/books/NBK8618/.

[6] Jackson AC. Rabies virus infection: An update. Journal of NeuroVirology. 2003;9(2):253-258.

[7] Ghosh JB, Roy M, Lahiri K, Bala AK. Acute flaccid paralysis due to rabies. Journal of pediatric neurosciences. 2009;4(1):33-35.

[8] Hemachudha T, Ugolini G, Wacharapluesadee S, Sungkarat W, Shuangshoti S, Laothamatas J. Human rabies: neuropathogenesis, diagnosis, and management. The Lancet Neurology. 2013;12(5):498-513.

[9] Suraweera W, Morris SK, Kumar R, Warrell DA, Warrell MJ, Jha P, et al. Deaths from Symptomatically Identifiable Furious Rabies in India: A Nationally Representative Mortality Survey. PLOS Neglected Tropical Diseases. 2012;6(10):e1847.

[10] Pleasure SJ, Fischbein NJ. Correlation of Clinical and Neuroimaging Findings in a Case of Rabies Encephalitis. Archives of Neurology. 2000;57(12):1765-1769.

[11] Laothamatas J, Sungkarat W, Hemachudha T. Chapter 14 - Neuroimaging in Rabies. In: Jackson AC, editor. Advances in Virus Research. 79: Academic Press; 2011. p. 309-27.

[12] Robardet E, Picard-Meyer E, Andrieu S, Servat A, Cliquet F. International interlaboratory trials on rabies diagnosis: An overview of results and variation in reference diagnosis techniques (fluorescent antibody test, rabies tissue culture infection test, mouse inoculation test) and molecular biology techniques. Journal of Virological Methods. 2011;177(1):15-25.

[13] Cliquet F, Aubert M, Sagné L. Development of a fluorescent antibody virus neutralisation test (FAVN test) for the quantitation of rabies-neutralising antibody. Journal of Immunological Methods. 1998;212(1):79-87.

[14] Prevention CfDCa, (NCEZID) NCfEaZID, (DHCPP) DoH-CPaP. Direct fluorescent antibody test: Centers for Disease Control and Prevention; 2011 [Available from: https://www.cdc.gov/rabies/diagnosis/direct_fluorescent_antibody.html.

[15] Centers for Disease Control and Prevention NCfEaZIDN, Division of High-Consequence Pathogens and Pathology (DHCPP). Rabies [Internet]. Centers for Disease Control and Prevention; 2020 [updated September 25, 2020. Available from: https://www.cdc.gov/rabies/index.html.

[16] Lembo T, Niezgoda M, Velasco-Villa A, Cleaveland S, Ernest E, Rupprecht CE. Evaluation of a direct, rapid immunohistochemical test for rabies diagnosis. Emerging infectious diseases. 2006;12(2):310-313.

[17] Matsumoto S. Electron microscopy of nerve cells infected with street rabies virus. Virology. 1962;17(1):198-202.

[18] David D, Yakobson B, Rotenberg D, Dveres N, Davidson I, Stram Y. Rabies virus detection by RT-PCR in decomposed naturally infected brains. Veterinary Microbiology. 2002;87(2): 111-118.

[19] Goswami U Fau - Shankar SK, Shankar Sk Fau - Channabasavanna SM, Channabasavanna Sm Fau - Chattopadhyay A, Chattopadhyay A. Psychiatric presentations in rabies. A clinico-pathologic report from South India with a review of literature. (0041-3232 (Print)).

[20] Bidaki R, Mirhosseini Mm, Asad F. Rabies or a psychiatric disorder? A rare case report. Neuropsychiatrie de l'Enfance et de l'Adolescence. 2013;60.

[21] Fishbain DA, Barsky S, Goldberg M. Monosymptomatic Hypochondriacal Psychosis: Belief of Contracting Rabies. The International Journal of Psychiatry in Medicine. 1992;22(1):3-9.

[22] Hampson K, Dushoff J, Cleaveland S, Haydon DT, Kaare M, Packer C, et al. Transmission Dynamics and Prospects for the Elimination of Canine Rabies. PLOS Biology. 2009;7(3):e1000053.

[23] Bronnert J, Wilde H, Tepsumethanon V, Lumlertdacha B, Hemachudha T. Organ Transplantations and Rabies Transmission. Journal of Travel Medicine. 2007;14(3):177-180.

[24] Winkler WG, Fashinell TR, Leffingwell L, Howard P, Conomy JP. Airborne Rabies Transmission in a Laboratory Worker. JAMA. 1973;226(10):1219-1221.

[25] Burton EC, Burns Dk Fau - Opatowsky MJ, Opatowsky Mj Fau - El-Feky WH, El-Feky Wh Fau - Fischbach B, Fischbach B Fau - Melton L, Melton L Fau - Sanchez E, et al. Rabies encephalomyelitis: clinical, neuroradiological, and pathological findings in 4 transplant recipients. (0003-9942 (Print)).

[26] Jackson AC, Warrell MJ, Rupprecht CE, Ertl HCJ, Dietzschold B, O'Reilly M, et al. Management of Rabies in Humans. Clinical Infectious Diseases. 2003;36(1):60-63.

[27] Hemachudha T, Laothamatas J, Rupprecht CE. Human rabies: a disease of complex neuropathogenetic mechanisms and diagnostic challenges. The Lancet Neurology. 2002;1(2): 101-109.

[28] Charlton KM, Nadin-Davis S Fau - Casey GA, Casey Ga Fau - Wandeler AI, Wandeler AI. The long incubation period in rabies: delayed progression of infection in muscle at the site of exposure. (0001-6322 (Print)).

[29] Marquette C, Van Dam A-M, Ceccaldi P-E, Weber P, Haour F, Tsiang H. Induction of immunoreactive interleukin-1β and tumor necrosis factor-α in the brains of rabies virus infected rats. Journal of Neuroimmunology. 1996;68(1):45-51.

[30] Appolin?rio CM, Allendorf SD, Peres MG, Ribeiro BD, Fonseca CvR, Vicente AcF, et al. Profile of Cytokines and Chemokines Triggered by Wild-Type Strains of Rabies Virus in Mice. The American Society of Tropical Medicine and Hygiene. 2016;94(2): 378-383.

[31] Chopy D, Detje Cn Fau - Lafage M, Lafage M Fau - Kalinke U, Kalinke U

Fau - Lafon M, Lafon M. The type I interferon response bridles rabies virus infection and reduces pathogenicity. (1538-2443 (Electronic)).

[32] Wang Z, Liang Q, Zhang Y, Yang J, Li M, Wang K, et al. An optimized HMGB1 expressed by recombinant rabies virus enhances immunogenicity through activation of dendritic cells in mice. Oncotarget. 2017;8(48): 83539-83554.

[33] Chen T, Zhang Y, Wang Z, Yang J, Li M, Wang K, et al. Recombinant rabies virus expressing IL-15 enhances immunogenicity through promoting the activation of dendritic cells in mice. Virologica Sinica. 2017;32(4):317-327.

[34] Tarantola A. Four Thousand Years of Concepts Relating to Rabies in Animals and Humans, Its Prevention and Its Cure. Tropical medicine and infectious disease. 2017;2(2):5.

[35] Organization WH. Frequently asked questions about rabies for the General Public [PDF]. 2018 [Available from: https://www.who.int/rabies/Rabies_General_Public_FAQs_21Sep2018.pdf.

[36] Hicks DJ, Fooks AR, Johnson N. Developments in rabies vaccines. Clinical and experimental immunology. 2012;169(3):199-204.

[37] Wu X, Smith T, Rupprecht C. From brain passage to cell adaptation: The road of human rabies vaccine development. Expert review of vaccines. 2011;10:1597-1608.

[38] Almeida RG, Pan S, Cole KLH, Williamson JM, Early JJ, Czopka T, et al. Myelination of Neuronal Cell Bodies when Myelin Supply Exceeds Axonal Demand. Current Biology. 2018;28(8):1296-305.e5.

[39] Koprowski H Fau - Cox HR, Cox HR. Studies on chick embryo adapted rabies virus; culture characteristics and pathogenicity. (0022-1767 (Print)).

[40] Madhusudana SN, Mani RS. Intradermal vaccination for rabies prophylaxis: conceptualization, evolution, present status and future. (1744-8395 (Electronic)).

[41] World Health Organization = Organisation mondiale de la S. Weekly Epidemiological Record, 2018, vol. 93, 16 [full issue]. Weekly Epidemio logical Record = Relevé épidémiologique hebdomadaire. 2018;93(16):201-20.

[42] Matson MA, Schenker E, Stein M, Zamfirova V, Nguyen H-B, Bergman GE. Safety and efficacy results of simulated post-exposure prophylaxis with human immune globulin (HRIG; KEDRAB) co-administered with active vaccine in healthy subjects: a comparative phase 2/3 trial. Human Vaccines & Immunotherapeutics. 2020;16(2): 452-459.

[43] Aoki FY, Rubin Me Fau - Friesen AD, Friesen Ad Fau - Bowman JM, Bowman Jm Fau - Saunders JR, Saunders JR. Intravenous human rabies immunoglobulin for post-exposure prophylaxis: serum rabies neutralizing antibody concentrations and side-effects. (0092-1157 (Print)).

[44] Bharti OK, Madhusudana SN, Wilde H. Injecting rabies immunoglobulin (RIG) into wounds only: A significant saving of lives and costly RIG. Human vaccines & immunotherapeutics. 2017;13(4): 762-765.

[45] Goudsmit J, Marissen We Fau - Weldon WC, Weldon Wc Fau - Niezgoda M, Niezgoda M Fau - Hanlon CA, Hanlon Ca Fau - Rice AB, Rice Ab Fau - Kruif Jd, et al. Comparison of an anti-rabies human monoclonal antibody combination with

human polyclonal anti-rabies immune globulin. (0022-1899 (Print)).

[46] Sparrow E, Torvaldsen S, Newall AT, Wood JG, Sheikh M, Kieny MP, et al. Recent advances in the development of monoclonal antibodies for rabies post exposure prophylaxis: A review of the current status of the clinical development pipeline. Vaccine. 2019;37:A132-A1A9.

[47] Willoughby RE, Tieves KS, Hoffman GM, Ghanayem NS, Amlie-Lefond CM, Schwabe MJ, et al. Survival after Treatment of Rabies with Induction of Coma. New England Journal of Medicine. 2005;352(24): 2508-2514.

[48] van Thiel P-PAM, de Bie RMA, Eftimov F, Tepaske R, Zaaijer HL, van Doornum GJJ, et al. Fatal Human Rabies due to Duvenhage Virus from a Bat in Kenya: Failure of Treatment with Coma-Induction, Ketamine, and Antiviral Drugs. PLOS Neglected Tropical Diseases. 2009;3(7):e428.

[49] Hemachudha T, Sunsanee witayakul B, Desudchit T, Suankratay C, Sittipunt C, Wacharapluesadee S, et al. Failure of therapeutic coma and ketamine for therapy of human rabies. Journal of neurovirology. 2006;12: 407-409.

[50] Jochmans D, Neyts J. The path towards effective antivirals against rabies. Vaccine. 2019;37(33): 4660-4662.

[51] Appolinário C, Jackson A. Antiviral therapy for human rabies. Antiviral therapy. 2014;20.

[52] Niu X, Tang L, Tseggai T, Guo Y, Fu ZF. Wild-type rabies virus phosphoprotein is associated with viral sensitivity to type I interferon treatment. Archives of Virology. 2013;158(11):2297-2305.

[53] Weinmann E Fau - Majer M, Majer M Fau - Hilfenhaus J, Hilfenhaus J. Intramuscular and/or intralumbar postexposure treatment of rabies virus-infected cynomolgus monkeys with human interferon. (0019-9567 (Print)).

[54] Merigan Tc Fau - Baer GM, Baer Gm Fau - Winkler WG, Winkler Wg Fau - Bernard KW, Bernard Kw Fau - Gibert CG, Gibert Cg Fau - Chany C, Chany C Fau - Veronesi R, et al. Human leukocyte interferon administration to patients with symptomatic and suspected rabies. (0364-5134 (Print)).

[55] Lockhart BP, Tsiang H, Ceccaldi PE, Guillemer S. Ketamine-Mediated Inhibition of Rabies Virus Infection in vitro and in Rat Brain. Antiviral Chemistry and Chemotherapy. 1991;2(1):9-15.

[56] Weli SC, Scott CA, Ward CA, Jackson AC. Rabies virus infection of primary neuronal cultures and adult mice: failure to demonstrate evidence of excitotoxicity. Journal of virology. 2006;80(20):10270-10273.

[57] Superti F Fau - Seganti L, Seganti L Fau - Panà A, Panà A Fau - Orsi N, Orsi N. Effect of amantadine on rhabdovirus infection. (0378-6501 (Print)).

[58] Jackson AC. Is minocycline useful for therapy of acute viral encephalitis? (1872-9096 (Electronic)).

[59] Jackson AC, Scott CA, Owen J, Weli SC, Rossiter JP. Therapy with minocycline aggravates experimental rabies in mice. Journal of virology. 2007;81(12):6248-6253.

[60] Yamada K, Noguchi K, Komeno T, Furuta Y, Nishizono A. Efficacy of Favipiravir (T-705) in Rabies Postexposure Prophylaxis. The Journal of Infectious Diseases. 2016;213(8): 1253-1261.

[61] Warrell M, Warrell DA, Tarantola A. The Imperative of Palliation in the Management of Rabies Encepha lomyelitis. Tropical medicine and infectious disease. 2017;2(4):52.

[62] Warrell DA. The clinical picture of rabies in man. Transactions of The Royal Society of Tropical Medicine and Hygiene. 1976;70(3):188-195.

[63] Goyal K, Garg N, Bithal P. Central fever: a challenging clinical entity in neurocritical care. J Neurocrit Care. 2020;13(1):19-31.

[64] Tarantola A, Crabol Y, Mahendra BJ, In S, Barennes H, Bourhy H, et al. Caring for patients with rabies in developing countries - the neglected importance of palliative care. (1365-3156 (Electronic)).

[65] World Health O, Food and Agriculture Organization of the United N, World Organisation for Animal H. Zero by 30: the global strategic plan to end human deaths from dog-mediated rabies by 2030. Geneva: World Health Organization; 2018 2018.

[66] Organization PAH, Center PAF-a-MD, Unit VPH. 14th Meeting of Directors of National Programs for Rabies Control in Latin America (REDIPRA). Lima, Peru; 2013.

[67] Nations FaAOotU, Control GAfR, Organization WH. The Stepwise Approach towards Rabies Elimination: A Planning and Evaluation Tool: Partners for Rabies Prevention; 2017 [Available from: https:// caninerabiesblueprint.org/IMG/pdf/ sare_outline_2017_f.pdf.

[68] Freuling CM, Hampson K, Selhorst T, Schröder R, Meslin FX, Mettenleiter TC, et al. The elimination of fox rabies from Europe: determinants of success and lessons for the future. Philosophical transactions of the Royal Society of London Series B, Biological sciences. 2013;368(1623):20120142.

Section 2

Epidemiology of the Rabies Virus - Practical Experience

Chapter 4

Occurrence of Dog Bites and Rabies within Humans in Srinagar, Kashmir

Namera Thahaby, Afzal Hoque Akand, Abdul Hai Bhat,
Shabeer Ahmed Hamdani and Mudasir Ali Rather

Abstract

Open garbage dumps and dog bites are major public health problems in the Kashmir region. In Srinagar city, there are more than 91,000 dogs, or about one dog for every 12 citizens. The mounting street dog population is leading to increasing fright in the city due to the fear of rabies. Although treatable, rabies can be deadly without access to vaccines and treatment. Unfortunately, Kashmir is experiencing a shortage of the anti-rabies vaccine. More than 80,000 dog bites and 20 deaths due to rabies were reported in the Kashmir valley in the period 2008–2012. We conducted our study of dog bites in Srinagar, which has a large stray dog population, perhaps due to mismanagement of garbage. We obtained our data from Shri Maharaja Hari Singh (SMHS) Hospital. We found that most dog bite victims were males aged 30–40 years presenting with category 3 bites to the legs. The majority of victims were bitten in the evening and reported to the hospital the same day. Most victims received immunoglobin treatment. We suggest that proper garbage control can help to curb the stray dog population in the area and thus reduce the incidence of rabies.

Keywords: rabies, dog bites, Srinagar, Kashmir

1. Introduction

Open garbage dumps and dog bites are major public health problems in the Kashmir region. In Srinagar city, there are more than 91,000 dogs [1], or about one dog for every 12 citizens. More than 80,000 dog bites and 20 deaths due to rabies were reported in the Kashmir valley in the period 2008–2012 [2]. The area's Anti-Rabies Clinic (ARC), Shri Maharaja Hari Singh (SMHS) Hospital, depleted its stock of vaccine fourfold in a ten-month period [3]. The overwhelming majority of dog bite cases (9514) occurred in Srinagar [4]. Of these cases, 80% occurred in urban spaces and 20% occurred in rural areas.

2. Research methodology

The present study was conducted in the Srinagar district in Kashmir, which has a large stray dog population, perhaps due to mismanagement of garbage. We obtained data on dog bites and victims from SMHS.

Wards	North zone (9 wards)	South zone (9 wards)	East zone (8 wards)	West zone (8 wards)
1	Tarbal, JamiaMasjid, Kawdara	Malroo, Lawaypora	Harwan, Nishat	SafaKadal, IddGah
2	Zadibal, Madeen Sahib	BeminaKhumaniChowk	Dalgate, Lalchowk	Palpora
3	Lal Bazaar, Umer Colony	AllochiBagh, MagermalBagh	Dud Dal, Locut dal	Nawab Bazaar, Ali Kadal
4	Hazratbal, Tailbal	Rajbagh, JawaharNagar, WazirBagh	JogiLankar, Zindashah Sahib	Syed Ali Akbar, Islam Yarbal
5	New Theed, Alusteng	Mahjoor Nagar, Natipora, Chanapora	Ganpatyar, Barbarshah	Shaheed Gung, Karan Nagar
6	Zakoora	BaghatBarzallua, Rawalpora	BanaMohalla,Chinkral Mohalla, S.R.Gung	Qamarwari, Chattabal
7	Ahmad Nagar	Humhama	Akil Mir Khanyar, Khaja Bazar	Bemina East, BeminaWest
8	Soura, Buchpora	PanthaChowk, Khanmoh	Hasna Abad, Makhdoom Sahib	Parimpora, Zainakote
9	Nowshahra, Zoonimar	S.D.colony Batamaloo Nundrash colony		

Table 1.
Srinagar Municipal Corporation zones and wards.

We categorized the incidents into zones as per the Srinagar Municipal Corporation, as shown in **Table 1**. This was done to determine which zone recorded the greatest number of cases.

3. Results

Table 2 shows the distribution of dog bite victims according to gender and zones (**Figure 1**). Overwhelmingly, the majority of victims in each zone are male. In the east zone, 82.23% of victims were males and 17.76% of victims were females. In the west zone, 71.90%, of victims were males and 28.09% of victims were females. In the north zone, 75.94% of victims were males and 27.05% of victims were females. In the south zone, 73.06% of victims were males and 26.93% of victims were females. Statistically, there is a nonsignificant difference concerning gender for

Gender	Zones			
	East	West	North	South
Male	162 (82.23)	238 (71.90)	213 (72.94)	236 (73.06)
Female	35 (17.76)	93 (28.09)	79 (27.05)	87 (26.93)
Pooled	197	331	292	323
	χ^2 = 8.023, p = 0.045			

Figures in parentheses indicate percentage.
*indicates difference at 5% level of significance.

Table 2.
Distribution of victims according to gender and zone.

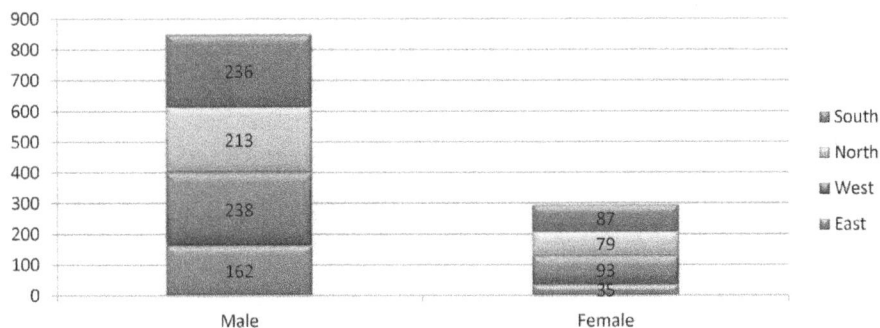

Figure 1.
Distribution of dog bite victims according to gender and zone.

different zones. **Table 3** shows the distribution of victim age according to zones. In the east zone, 24.87%, of victims were aged 30–40 years, 19.28% of victims were aged 20–30 years, 14.72% were aged 10–20 years, 12.89% were aged 40–50 years, 12.69% were aged 1–10 years, 9.64% were aged 50–60 years, and the remaining 6.59% of victims were aged 60 years and older.

The same pattern was observed for the west, north, and south zones. Statistically, there is a nonsignificant difference concerning age for different zones. **Table 4** shows the date of reporting according to different zones. In the east zone, 67.51% of victims reported on the same day, 25.88% reported after a day or more, and the remaining 6.59% reported after a week. The same pattern was observed among the other zones. Statistically, there was a nonsignificant difference concerning the date of reporting for different zones. **Table 5** depicts the distribution of victims according to the time of exposure for different zones. In the east zone, 53.80% of victims were bitten by dogs in the evening, 29.44% were bitten in the morning, 8.62% were bitten in the daytime, and 8.12% were bitten in the nighttime. The same pattern was again seen in the other zones. Statistically, there was a nonsignificant difference concerning the time of exposure for different zones. **Table 6** depicts victims according to the time of reporting for different zones. In the

Age	Zones			
	East	West	North	South
1–10 years	25 (12.69)	33 (9.96)	33 (11.30)	39 (12.07)
10–20 years	29 (14.72)	43 (12.29)	43 (14.72)	58 (17.95)
20–30 years	38 (19.28)	63 (19.03)	58 (19.86)	64 (19.81)
30–40 years	49 (24.87)	102 (30.81)	84 (28.76)	70 (21.69)
40–50 years	24 (12.18)	44 (13.29)	32 (10.95)	45 (13.93)
50–60 years	19 (9.64)	31 (9.36)	22 (7.53)	22 (6.81)
60 years and older	13 (6.59)	15 (4.53)	20 (6.84)	25 (7.73)
Pooled	197	331	292	323
Mean SD	33.91 17.49	47.28 28.22	41.7 22.6	46.14 18.75
	χ^2 = 15.726, p = 0.611			

Figures in parentheses indicate percentage.
*indicates difference at 5% level of significance.

Table 3.
Distribution of dog bite victims according to age and zone.

Date of reporting	Zones			
	East	West	North	South
Same day	133 (67.51)	255 (77.03)	221 (75.68)	261 (80.80)
After one day or more	51 (25.88)	63 (19.03)	55 (18.83)	45 (13.93)
After a week	13 (6.59)	13 (3.92)	16 (5.47)	17 (5.26)
Pooled	197	331	292	323

$\chi^2 = 14.103$, p = 0.028

Figures in parentheses indicate percentage.
*indicates difference at 5% level of significance.

Table 4.
Distribution of dog bite victims according to date of reporting and zone.

Time of exposure	Zones			
	East	West	North	South
Morning	58 (29.44)	86 (25.98)	63 (21.57)	55 (17.02)
Daytime	17 (8.62)	28 (8.45)	29 (9.93)	29 (8.97)
Evening	106 (53.80)	203 (61.32)	183 (62.67)	227 (70.27)
Night	16 (8.12)	14 (4.22)	17 (5.82)	12 (3.71)
Pooled	197	331	292	323

$\chi^2 = 21.524$, p = 0.01

Figures in parentheses indicate percentage.
*indicates difference at 5% level of significance.

Table 5.
Distribution of dog bite victims according to time of exposure and zone.

Time of reporting	Zones			
	East	West	North	South
Morning	72 (36.54)	98 (29.60)	85 (29.10)	83 (25.69)
Day	28 (14.21)	54 (16.31)	44 (15.06)	46 (14.24)
Evening	84 (42.63)	165 (49.84)	153 (52.39)	179 (55.41)
Night	13 (6.59)	14 (4.22)	10 (3.42)	15 (4.64)
Pooled	197	331	292	323

$\chi^2 = 12.34$, p = 0.194

Figures in parentheses indicate percentage.
*indicates difference at 5% level of significance.

Table 6.
Distribution of dog bite victims according to time of reporting and zone.

east zone, 42.63% victims reported in the evening, 36.54% reported in the morning, 14.21% reported in the daytime, and 6.59% reported in the nighttime. **Table 7** depicts victims according to the site of the bite. In the east zone, 63.45% of victims had bites on the legs, 13.19% had bites on the hands, arms, and shoulders, 7.01% had bites on the buttocks, 13.19% had bites on the knees and thighs, 1.01% had bites on the face, and 2.03% had bites on the abdomen and back. Likewise, the other zones

Site of bite	Zones			
	East	West	North	South
Face	2 (1.01)	7 (2.11)	3 (1.02)	7 (2.16)
Hands, arms, & shoulders	26 (13.19)	75 (22.65)	65 (22.26)	70 (21.67)
Legs	125 (63.45)	173 (52.26)	159 (54.45)	190 (58.82)
Knees, thighs	26 (13.19)	31 (9.36)	25 (8.56)	22 (6.81)
Buttocks	14 (7.10)	36 (10.87)	33 (11.30)	30 (9.28)
Abdomen & back	4 (2.03)	9 (2.71)	7 (2.39)	4 (1.23)
Pooled	197	331	292	323
χ^2 = 21.899, p = 0.11				

Figures in parentheses indicate percentage.
*indicates difference at 5% level of significance.

Table 7.
Distribution of dog bite victims according to site of bite and zone.

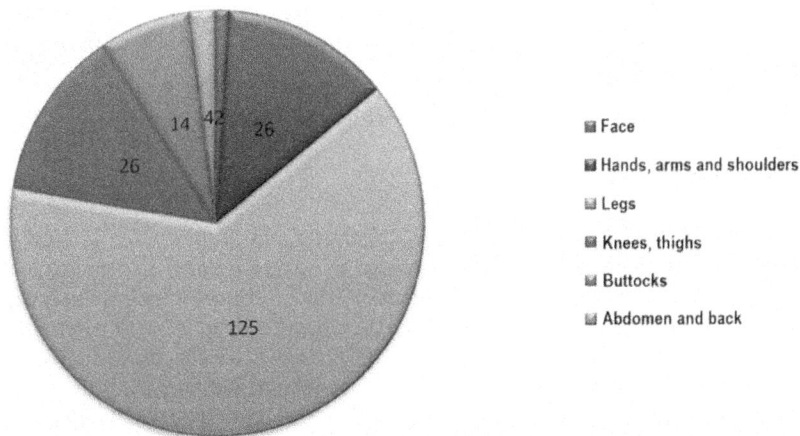

Figure 2.
Site of bite.

Category of bite	Zones			
	East	West	North	South
1	0 (0.00)	0 (0.00)	0 (0.00)	0 (0.00)
2	47 (23.85)	114 (34.44)	92 (31.50)	88 (27.24)
3	150 (76.14)	217 (65.55)	200 (68.49)	235 (72.75)
Pooled	197	331	292	323
Fisher exact test = 0.04*				

Figures in parentheses indicate percentage.
*indicates difference at 5% level of significance.

Table 8.
Distribution of dog bite victims according to category of bite and zone.

Immunoglobin	Zones			
	East	**West**	**North**	**South**
Received	153 (77.66)	266 (80.36)	246 (84.24)	282 (87.30)
Didn't receive	44 (22.33)	65 (19.63)	46 (15.75)	41 (12.69)
Pooled	197	331	292	323
	$\chi^2 = 10.085$, p = 0.017			

Figures in parentheses indicate percentage.
*indicates difference at 5% level of significance.

Table 9.
Distribution of dog bite victims who received immunoglobin treatment according to zone.

showed a similar trend. Statistically, there was a nonsignificant difference concerning the site of bite for different zones (**Figure 2**). **Table 8** depicts victims according to the category of bite. In the east zone, 76.14% of victims had category 3 bites, while 23.85% had category 2 bites. A similar pattern was observed for the other zones. **Table 9** depicts victims according to those who received immunoglobin treatment. In the east zone, 87.30% of victims received immunoglobin, while 12.69% did not. The other zones showed a similar distribution. Statistically, there was a nonsignificant difference in receiving immunoglobin for different zones.

4. Discussion

Rabies is a deadly disease if not treated promptly and properly. In our study, we collected data on dog bite victims and patterns in different zones in Srinagar, Kashmir. We found that males were bitten more than females, which is likely due to the fact that men in the area venture out of their homes to go to work more often than the women do. Most victims are 30 to 40 years old, which conforms with the findings of Mohammadzadeh et al. [5] and Agarvval and Reddaiah [6]. Due to fear of rabies, most victims reported to the hospital on the same day they were bitten. The highest number of cases was seen in the evening when people usually return from work and school. The site of the bite is important, as the rabies virus has broad tissue tropism. The majority of dog bites were to the legs, which other studies by Ain et al. [4], Acharya et al. [7], Chopra et al. [8], and Agarvval and Reddaiah [6] have also confirmed. When a dog threatens a person, it typically bites the lower extremities. Conversely, when a person threatens a dog, the dog is more prone to biting the upper extremities. Although only some of the bites were to the face and head, we observed that children aged younger than 10 years were more prone to being bitten on the head compared to older victims. Typically, children display offensive acts toward dogs, and the head of a child is closer to the mouth of a dog. Most of the bites were category 3, which means the bites penetrated the skin and caused deep wounds. Victims of category 3 bites received immunoglobin treatment. The west zone of the city experienced the greatest number of dog bite incidents. This might be because the area is crowded and has many open garbage dumps, which attract stray dogs and increase the risk of rabies transmission. The west zone is a downtown area where streets are densely inhabited and where people regularly throw food into the streets. The accessibility of food in the garbage not only augments fertility in dogs but also makes them more prone to attack humans whom they may view as competition for food.

5. Conclusion

Open garbage dumps are a public health problem and they have led to an increased stray dog population in Srinagar, Kashmir, and thus an increased incident of dog bites and rabies cases. We suggest that proper garbage control can help to curb the stray dog population in the area and thus reduce the incidence of rabies.

Abbreviations

SMHS   Shri Maharaja Hari Singh Hospital

Author details

Namera Thahaby[1*], Afzal Hoque Akand[1], Abdul Hai Bhat[1], Shabeer Ahmed Hamdani[1] and Mudasir Ali Rather[2]

1 Division of Veterinary and Animal Husbandry Extension, FVSc & AH, SKUAST-Kashmir, Srinagar, J&K, India

2 Division of Veterinary Public Health, FVSc & AH, SKUAST-Kashmir, Srinagar, J&K, India

*Address all correspondence to: nimrazahbi@gmail.com

IntechOpen

References

[1] Lone KS, Bilquees S, Khan MS, Haq IU. Analysis of dog bites in Kashmir: An unprovoked threat to human population. National Journal of Community Medicine. 2014;5(1):66-68

[2] The Greater Kashmir. (Hasan, 2013). Kashmir: 20 Rabies Deaths, 80,000 Dogs Bite Cases in 5 Years

[3] The Greater Kashmir. 2018. Acute shortage of Antirabies Vaccine Hits Hospital

[4] Ain SN, Khan SMS, Azhar M, Haq S, Bashir K. Epidemiological profile of animal bite victims attending an antirabies clinic in district Srinagar, Kashmir. Journal of Medical Sciences and Clinical Research. 2018;6:599-603

[5] Mohammadzadeh A, Mahmoodi P, Sharifi A, Moafi M, Erfani H, Siavashi M. A three-year epidemiological study of animal bites and rabies in Hamadan Province of Iran. Avicenna Journal of Clinical Microbial Infection. 2017;4(2):1-2

[6] Agarvval N, Reddaiah VP. Knowledge, attitude and practices following dog bite a community based epidemiology study. Health and Population: Perspectives and Issues. 2003;26:159-161

[7] Acharya R, Sethia R, Sharma G, Meena R. An analysis of animal bite cases attending anti rabies clinic attached to tertiary care center, Bikaner, Rajasthan, India. International Journal of Community Medicine Public Health. 2016;3(7):1945-1948

[8] Chopra D, Jauhari N, Dhungana H, Nasrah. Assessment of awareness about rabies and the animal bite among the staff nurses in a medical institute in Lucknow. International Journal of Community Medicine and Public Health. 2017;4(6):2046-2051

Chapter 5

Rabies Virus Infection in Livestock

Abdelmalik I. Khalafalla and Yahia H. Ali

Abstract

Rabies is a lethal zoonotic encephalomyelitis and a major challenge to public and animal health. Livestock are affected by rabies mostly through bites of rapid dogs or wildlife carnivore's species. They are considered as 'dead-end' hosts that do not transmit the virus. Rabies in livestock has been endemic in many developing countries for many years and diagnosed through clinical signs and dog-biting history. An introduction on rabies situation in farm animals will be given then subchapters including `rabies in bovines, rabies in small ruminants, rabies in swine and rabies in camelids. In each subchapter we shall discuss, epidemiology, modes of transmission, diagnosis and prevention and control measures.

Keywords: rabies, old world camelids, new world camelids, epidemiology, diagnosis, spread

1. Introduction

Rabies is the oldest known zoonotic fatal viral disease that affects only warm-blooded mammals. The rabies virus (RABV) infects the central nervous system transmitted through direct contact (such as through broken skin or mucous membranes in the eyes, nose, or mouth) with saliva or brain/nervous system tissue by an infected animal.

RABV almost exclusively infects neurons and eventually causing disease in the brain and death. The virus particle binds cell-surface receptors and follows the endosomal pathway. The virus's life cycle then advances, and following several days or months, the virus enters the peripheral nerves (**Figure 1**). It is then transported to the central nervous system by retrograde flow in the axons [1].

People usually get rabies from the bite of a rabid animal. Around 99% of human cases of rabies are due to dog bites or rarely from non-bite exposures, which include scratches, abrasions, or open wounds. RABV can infect any mammal. However, animal species reported to be involved in the transmission of rabies to domestic farm animals are dogs, foxes, wolves, jackals, and vampire bats (**Figure 2**).

The species of livestock and the carnivores that transmit RABV to them vary from geographical area to another. For instance, according to Kasem et al. (2019), camels, sheep and goats are the most affected species among farm animals by rabies (21.5%, 16.5%, and 16.5%, respectively) and foxes and wolves (11.4% and 2.5%, respectively) are the most common wild animals infected with rabies in Saudi Arabia (**Figure 3**). **Table 1** show reported animal rabies cases according to the reviewed articles in some Asian, African, European, and Latin American countries.

The circulation of rabies virus among livestock has extraordinarily influenced endeavors to control the disease in humans as these animals are in regular contact

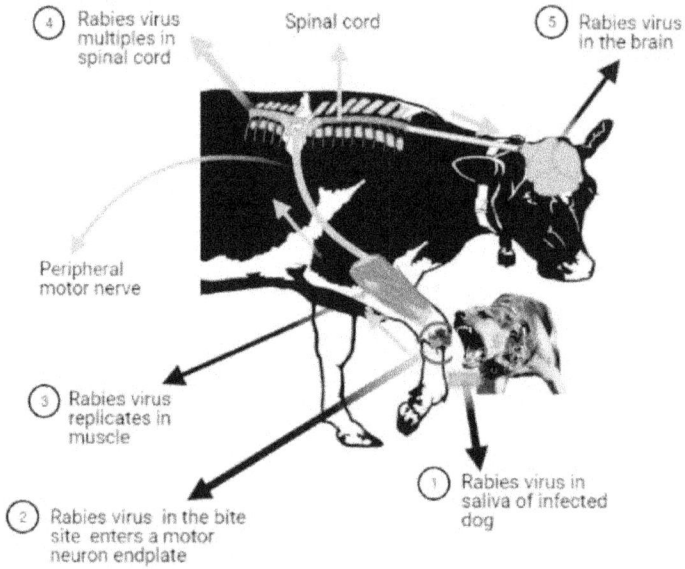

Figure 1.
Pathogenesis and spread of rabies virus in animals from the bite site to the central nervous system.

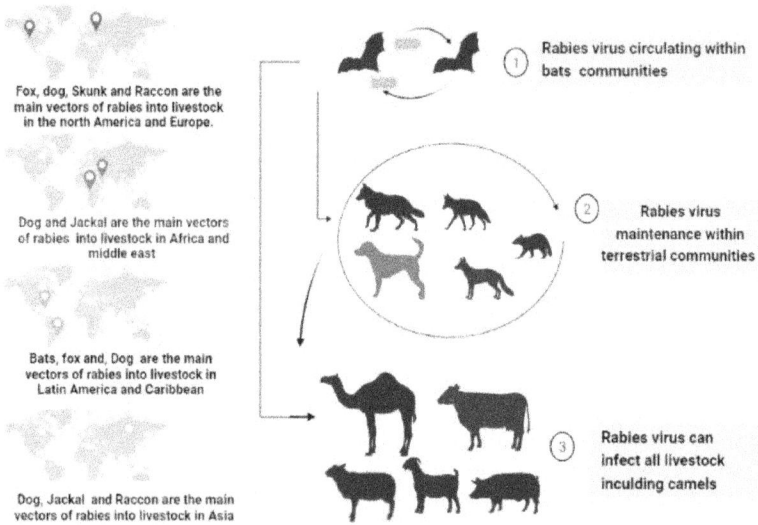

Figure 2.
Rabies virus transmission cycle in bats, terrestrial animals, and livestock.

with individuals. Additionally, affected livestock pose a potential risk to veterinarians and farmers, which underline the importance of applying rabies control measures to humans [15]. Rabies is a transmissible disease among animals causing economic losses directly or indirectly on the local and national economy. Due to their total reliance on livestock for their livelihoods, the losses due to rabies are relatively high for pastoral peoples in rural areas of the world due to their total dependence on livestock. Nevertheless, rabies in livestock remains underreported in developing countries because most of these countries lack adequate and efficient reporting systems and only clinical diagnosis is accessible.

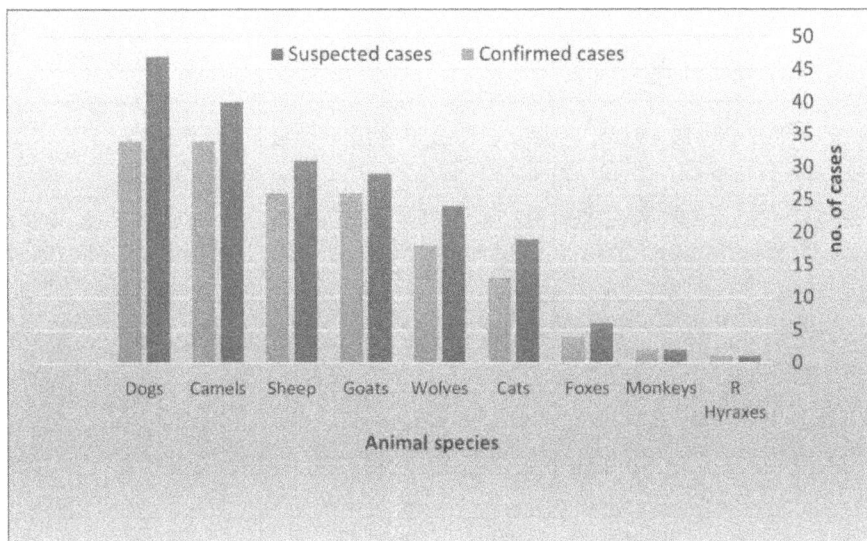

Figure 3.
*Suspected and confirmed cases of rabies in animals in Saudi Arabia recorded between 2010 and 2017 (modified from **Table 1** in Kasem et al. [15].*

2. Economic impact of rabies in livestock

Hampson et al. [38] estimated the economic costs of canine rabies to be 8.6 billion USD, mainly due to loss of productivity due to premature deaths, costs of post-exposure prophylaxis (PEP), and income loss for seeking PEP. Costs of Livestock deaths were 512 million USD per year, especially in livestock-dependent African economies (e.g., Sudan, Ethiopia, and Tanzania) and Asia (China, India, Bangladesh, and Pakistan). In Bhutan, rabies results in loss of cattle and their production, thus causing direct economic losses to the farmers besides a cost to the government due to managing outbreaks and provision of mass rabies PEP [39]. Most rabies human deaths were in Asia and Africa. Estimated rabies human deaths worldwide annually are 55,000, about 31,000 in Asia and 24,000 in Africa. In Bangladesh, dogs bit nearly 100,000 people, with at least 2,000 rabies deaths in 2009 [40].

Besides its public health significance, the occurrence of rabies in domestic animals (cattle, sheep, and goats), which are the source of food and income to the poor rural people, had raised its economic importance. The authors reviewed a report stating that the incidence of rabies in livestock is re-emerging disease reported in rabies endemic and free countries [29].

3. Laboratory diagnosis of rabies in livestock

During the eclipse phase after infection, the rabies virus replicates in non-nervous tissue such as muscle. After several days or months, the virus enters the peripheral nerves and is transported to the central nervous system and then disseminated within the CNS and the highly innervated tissues, resulting in clinical signs. Most of the virus is found in nervous tissue, salivary glands, saliva, and cerebrospinal fluid (CSF), which should all be handled with extreme caution. As there are neither gross pathognomonic lesions nor specific and constant

Country	Animal species								Reference
	Dog	Cattle	Goat	Sheep	Equidae	Camel	Pig	Fox	
Bangladesh		10	1		1 (Horse)				Uddin et al. [2]
	384	290	355						Islam et al. [3]
India						1			Kumar and Jindal [4]
							3		Preethi et al. [5]
Sri-Lanka	6788	915	233	13					Pushpakumara et al. [6]
China							20		Jiang et al. [7]
		21				15			Liu et al. [8]
				36					Zhu et al. [9]
Nepal	374	442	122	60	14 (Horses)		21		Devleesschauwer et al. (2016)
Iran		6							Simani et al. [10]
Jordan						12			Mohammadpour et al. [11]
						8			Al-Rawashdeh et al. [12]
Oman	2		312*			40		47	Al-Abaidani et al. (2015)
						22			Ahmed et al. [13]
Indonesia (Bali)	7114	8	1				1		Putra [14]
Saudi Arabia	34		26	26		34		18	Kasem et al. [15]
Uganda	15	6	4					1	Omodo et al. [16]

Country	Animal species								Reference
	Dog	Cattle	Goat	Sheep	Equidae	Camel	Pig	Fox	
Sudan	1158					83			Ali et al. (2004)
		172	501	82	33 (Horses), 467 (Donkeys)	79			Ali, et al. [17]
	708	76	184	111	12 (Horses), 277 (Donkeys)	60			Ali, et al. (2009)
	64	53	34	28	26 (Horses)	11			Baraa et al. [18],
						5			Abbas and Omer [19],
		1	1			6			Ahmed et al. [20],
	4	1	1		4 (Donkeys)				Ali [21]
Ethiopia	1951								Nibret [22]
	1434								Reta, et al. [23]
	1724	37			13 (Horses), 19 Donkey				Oyda and Megersa [24]
		28	12	5	3 (Horses)				Mulugeta et al. [25]
Kenya	2796	1192	280 (sheep & goat)		113	1		17	Bitek et al. [26]
Morocco	2458	2390	331 (sheep & goat)		1455 (Horses)	9			Darkaoui et al. [27]
Algeria	667	98							Matter et al. (2015)
Nigeria			1						Kaltungo et al. (2018)
		1							Ibrahim et al. [28]
		5	1	1					Tekki et al. [29]

Country	Animal species								Reference
	Dog	Cattle	Goat	Sheep	Equidae	Camel	Pig	Fox	
Sierra Leone		9							Suluku et al. [30]
Ghana							3		Tasiame et al. (2016)
Namibia	644	592	131						Hikufe et al. (2019)
USA	62	36	11*		13 (Horses)			314	Xiaoyue et al. (2018)
Brazil							2		Pessoa et al. [31]
			6						Moreira et al. [32]
Mexico		1037							Bárcenas-Reyes et al. [33]
Guatemala		154							Gilbert et al. [34]
Russian Federation	3731	6740						4347	Botvinkin and Kosenko [35]
Belarus	215	129						734	Botvinkin and Kosenko [35]
Latvia	566							2281	Westerling et al. [36]
Lithuania	183	638						802	Westerling et al. [36]
Estonia	131	81						566	Westerling et al. [36]
Ukraine	78	7	1		2			226	Polupan et al. [37]

*Both sheep and goats.

Table 1.
Reported animal rabies cases according to the reviewed articles in some Asian, African, European, and Latin American countries.

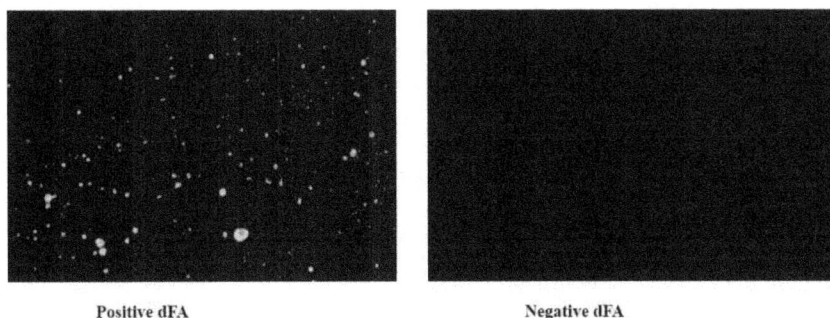

Positive dFA   Negative dFA

Figure 4.
Direct fluorescent antibody test (dFA), brain impression smears (source: Centers for Disease Control and Prevention (CDC)).

clinical signs for rabies, confirmatory laboratory diagnosis must be performed [41]. Laboratory diagnosis of rabies is based on the direct detection of rabies viral antigen using different histopathological and serological techniques with the dominance of fluorescent antibody test (FAT) (**Figure 4**). RABV infection induces the formation of cytosolic protein aggregates called Negri Bodies (NBs) detected by histopathology. However, this test is no longer recommended for diagnosis [41]. Brain samples are tested using the rapid immuno-chromatographic and direct Fluorescent Antibody assay in Nigeria [28, 29]. In China, FAT and RT/PCR are used for diagnosing rabies [8]. Real-time PCR is used as well in different laboratories [30]. Diagnosis of rabies is performed in Ethiopia by animal inoculation, cell cultures, serological tests, histological examination, molecular methods, and immunohistochemistry [42].

In Iran, laboratory diagnosis of rabies is practiced using different techniques, antigen in saliva using mouse inoculation test (MIT), fluorescence antibody test (FAT) and rapid tissue cell inoculation test (RTCIT). Antibodies against rabies in serum and cerebrospinal fluid (CSF) using mouse neutralization test (MNT) [10].

4. Prevention and control measures

It is important to remember that in developed countries, where canine rabies is eliminated, the virus may circulate in wildlife. In contrast, in most developing countries, the principal reservoir is dogs. The major rabies control strategies are vaccination of susceptible animals, mainly dogs and cats, elimination or control of stray dogs, and pre- and post-exposure vaccination of humans at risk. For rabies vaccination in animals, inactivated virus (for companion animals and livestock), live attenuated virus (for wildlife and free-roaming dogs), or recombinant vaccines (for wildlife, cats, and dogs) are used [41]. In China, local rabies vaccines have been used for emergency immunization of beef and dairy cattle and Bactrian (two-humped) camels [8]. In Ukraine, vaccination of domestic dogs and cats, besides oral vaccination of wild animals, mainly foxes, is adopted to control rabies [37]. In Latin America, due to attacks of bats, rabies is a significant problem, especially in cattle; many countries tend to vaccinate cattle but with an inadequate response from owners. In Guatemala, cattle vaccination coverage was estimated to be 11% [34]. In Latin America (e.g., Guatemala), vampire bat control activities (poisoning or culling) are used to control rabies in cattle, besides vaccination of cattle, although it is not widely used due to high cost [34]. In Morocco, free annual rabies vaccination campaigns for dogs are practiced; nevertheless, only around 6%

vaccination coverage rate is achieved. Elimination of stray dogs is done by shooting or using strychnine poison [43]. In Algeria, a mean of 131 positive dog rabies cases were reported annually; this is considered extremely high compared to neighboring Tunisia and Morocco. Elimination of stray dogs and vaccination of canines are the main control measures adopted [44].

Vaccination of livestock in affected areas was implemented in 2012 in Bela Vista city, Arkansas state, USA, where a rabies outbreak was reported. More than 200 cattle were vaccinated with two doses of the vaccine to prevent the disease in bovine, equine, goat, and sheep (reviewed by [29]).

5. Rabies in cattle

Cattle, like other warm-blooded animals, are susceptible to rabies infection. The incidence of rabies in cattle is variable according to the management system.

5.1 Epidemiology

The incidence of rabies in cattle is continuously reported worldwide. In India and Bangladesh, cattle were found to be the most affected domestic animals with rabies [2]. Cattle were the first most likely livestock tested positive for rabies in Mongolia [45]. Rabies was considered one of the most common infectious diseases affecting cattle and is most reported in cattle in Bhutan [39]. In Sri Lanka, cattle were the second most clinically diagnosed species with rabies during 2005–2014 [6]. In China, during 2004–2018, results of a rabies survey showed that cattle were the second most (12.5%) affected species according to rabies laboratory-confirmed cases [46]. In India, rabies' prevalence was 61.4% in cattle and buffalo [47]. In Nepal, cattle and buffalo appeared to be the most affected species even than dogs [48]. According to Bárcenas-Reyes et al. (2019), there is an increase in rabies cases in humans and cattle in Latin America and the Caribbean. Taghreed and Asmaa [49] reviewed some published rabies reports in Oman, Saudi Arabia, Egypt, Algeria, Iraq, and Yemen. Dogs were the main rabies reservoir, and the disease was found in camels, foxes, cattle, sheep, and goats. Dogs, cattle, and humans are the most common hosts for rabies in Ethiopia. Cattle come second to dogs [24]. Out of 48 animal deaths of rabies, cattle (28) were more affected than other animal species [25]. The same picture was reported in Nigeria [29]. In Kenya, cattle were found to be the second most rabies-affected species.

Within samples submitted for rabies diagnosis, those of cattle, goats, sheep, and horses showed a higher percentage of positivity than dog and cat ones [26]. In Namibia, cattle rabies cases are second to dogs during 2011–2017 [50], also in Uganda during 2011–2013 [16]. In South Africa, rabies has been mainly diagnosed in dogs (52%), followed by (34%) cattle [51]. In a review about rabies in Morocco, most of the reviewed reports showed that cattle were found to be the second most affected animal after dogs [27, 52].

In Euro-Asia and Europe, until 2001, cattle were the first rabies affected species in the Russian Federation, second in Belarus [35], the first one in Lithuania, the second one in Latvia, and the third after dogs and cats in Estonia [36]. In Guatemala, 154 cattle rabies due to vampire bat bites were reported (reviewed by [34]). In the United States, Canada, and Mexico, few cases were reported in cattle [53]. The same situation showing a very few reported rabies cases in cattle in Ukraine during 2012–2016 was reported [37].

5.2 Clinical signs

The paralytic form of rabies is the main sign in cattle, but some animals also show depression and excitation [54]. Foaming, bellowing, hitting and biting any object, hazing at humans and other cows were reported in Sierra Leone [30]. In Peru, abortive rabies cases were reported, rabies virus neutralizing antibodies were detected in 11% of cattle in areas of vampire bats, no deaths were observed in those animals within two years [55]. The observed clinical signs of rabies in cattle in two localities in India and Bangladesh were aggression, mania, profuse salivation, frenzy, and restlessness [2].

5.3 Transmission

Rabies virus is transmitted mainly through bites from rabid dogs, which accounts for over 90% of confirmed rabies cases [29]. However, according to Acha [56], rabies affecting bovines is primarily a problem of the southern area of the Hemisphere where vampire bats transmit it. In Africa, domestic dogs are the essential reservoir and transmitter of rabies to humans and other domestic animals [22, 57]. However, according to Warrell [58], jackals are the reservoir species in Botswana, Namibia, Zimbabwe, and bat-eared foxes in northern South Africa.

Rabies is transmitted to cattle mainly by the bite of rabid dogs in Bhutan [39]. In China, dogs are the primary transmitters, while in border areas, wild foxes are [46]; camels and wild foxes were reported to transmit rabies to cattle [8]. In Saudi Arabia, the main reservoirs of rabies are reported to be foxes and wild dogs [15].

In Europe, the increase in rabies cases in domestic animals like cattle, sheep, horses, cats, and dogs is associated with increased disease incidence in red foxes. Wild animals are reported as a cause for more than 90% of the animal rabies cases in the U.S. and Canada in 2010 [59]. Foxes are the main affected animals and the source of rabies infection in Ukraine [37]. In Latin America and the Caribbean, the main transmitter of rabies is the blood-sucking bat [33, 54]. In Colombia, the major transmitters, reservoirs, and vectors of the rabies are insectivorous, frugivorous and hematophagous bats; Vampire bat, which appeared as the main rabies reservoir from Mexico to South America [60].

Cattle can transmit rabies to humans as well as other animals. In Iran, a case of human rabies due to contact with the saliva of rabid cattle was reported [10].

6. Rabies in goats

6.1 Epidemiology

In Ethiopia, of 48 animal deaths of rabies, 12 were goats which were the second more affected animal species [25]. In Sudan, a review on rabies showed that goats were the most rabies-affected species after dogs, as clear from previous reports [17, 18, 61, 62]. In Kenya, the third most rabies-affected species were sheep and goats [26]. The same situation was reported in Morocco [27] and Namibia [50]. In South Africa, rabies-diagnosed cases in goats were the third-highest figures after dogs and cattle [51]. The same situation was reported in Uganda during 2011–2013 [16].

Reported dog bite in goats was higher than in cattle in Bangladesh [3]. The reported prevalence of rabies in goats in India was 48.7% [47]. Sheep and goats showed the third-highest positivity reported for rabies diagnosis in Oman [63]. In Saudi Arabia during 2010–2017, confirmed rabies cases in goats were the third-highest number following dogs and camels [15]. In Sri Lanka, goats were the third most species that clinically rabies diagnosed during 2005–2014 [6]. In Nepal, goats were the fourth most affected species [48]. However, Uddin et al. (2015) reported that goats showed a low level of rabies prevalence (0.5%) in Bangladesh.

Compared to other species, a low number of cases were reported in goats in United States, Canada, and Mexico [53]. A very few rabies cases in goats in Ukraine were reported during 2012–2016 [37]. Rabies virus neutralizing antibodies were detected in 5% of goats in areas of vampire bats in Peru, seropositive animals remained healthy for further two years suggesting abortive rabies infection [55].

6.2 Clinical signs

Uddin et al. (2015) reported that in Bangladesh, profuse salivation and restlessness were the only observed clinical signs of rabies in goats. The authors reviewed other reports describing salivation (16%) and restlessness (3%), others reporting 100% for salivation, behavioral change, or mania, 70% for aggression or hyperesthesia. In Nigeria, Restlessness, agitation, and aggression were observed in rabies-affected goats [29]. A paralytic form of rabies was reported in goats in Brazil [54]. The same picture was reported in Brazil, where six goats bitten by bats showed apathy, isolation from the herd, sternal and lateral recumbency. Previously reported clinical signs showed that the furious form of rabies is more commonly appears in goats, aggressiveness occurs in 83%, excessive bleating in 72%, salivation in 29%, and paralysis in 17% of cases (**Figure 5**) [32]. In Nigeria, a case of rabies in goat was presented with nibbling on the metal fence, foamy salivation, excessive bloating, and inability to eat or drink [64].

6.3 Transmission

Dogs are the primary rabies transmitter to goats; rabies reservoirs are variable in different countries. Canine rabies is dominant in Africa, Asia, the Middle East, and Latin America, where bats play an increasing role in the latter. In North America and Europe, canine rabies has been greatly eliminated; rabies is maintained in wildlife, as reviewed by Tilahun et al. [65]. In Bali, dogs are the primary source of rabies infection to human and domestic animals [14]. Most reported rabies cases in goats were due to dog attacks, especially in African and Asian countries [3, 16, 18, 21, 47]. Sheep and goats accounted for a meager percentage as a source of rabies infection for humans in Ethiopia [23].

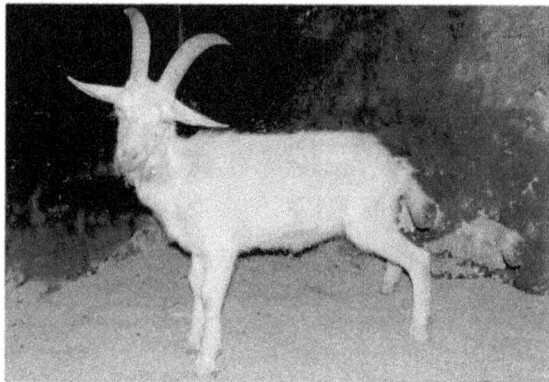

Figure 5.
Rabid Saanen buck presenting depression, somnolence and abnormal standing position (source: [32]).

7. Rabies in sheep

7.1 Epidemiology

In Kenya, sheep and goats were the third most rabies-affected species [26]. The same situation was reported in Morocco [27] and Namibia [50]. In South Africa, rabies diagnosed in sheep were the fourth-highest figures after dogs, cattle, and goats [51]. In Oman, sheep and goats showed the third-highest positivity reported for rabies diagnosis [63]. During 2004–2018 in China, it was noticed that sheep were the third most (9.7%) affected species [46]. Confirmed rabies in sheep was the third-highest number following dogs and camels in Saudi Arabia during 2010–2017 [15]. Within the affected species, a low number of cases was reported in sheep in United States, Canada, and Mexico [53].

7.2 Clinical signs

In sheep, attacking people and other animals besides other abnormal behavior was seen in Nigeria [29]. In Nigeria, observed clinical signs in a rabid ewe were aggressiveness, restlessness, corneal opacity, muscular tremor, hydrophobia, and salivation [57]. In an outbreak of rabies in sheep in China, clinical signs observed were arched back, tremors, and a swimming movement of all four limbs, followed by paralysis and death [9]. A paralytic form of rabies was reported in sheep in Brazil [54]. In another study in Brazil, clinical signs observed were abnormal gait, trembling, lateral recumbency, convulsion, opisthotonos, and fever [66]. Abortive rabies cases were reported in sheep in Peru, rabies virus neutralizing antibodies were detected in 3.6% of sheep that were healthy for two years later [55].

7.3 Transmission

The main transmitter of rabies to sheep is dogs. In Africa, the source of most rabies reported cases in sheep was the dog [29, 57, 62]. In China, dogs are the main rabies transmitters, while in border areas, wild foxes are [46]; wild foxes were reported to transmit rabies to sheep [8]. An increase in rabies cases in sheep is associated with a rise in the disease incidence in red foxes in Europe [59]. Rabies transmission from sheep to human was reported; three patients got rabies from direct contact with their sheep which a wolf had attacked in Iran [10].

8. Rabies in camelids

8.1 Epidemiology

Camelids are susceptible to rabies. However, most of the publications described clinical rabies in dromedary camels (*Camelus dromedarius*), with few reports in Bactrian camels (*Camelus bactrianus*) [8, 46] and the New World camelids [67]. From 2006 to 2013 in Oman, foxes reported the highest positivity rate (70.1%), camels accounted for the second higher positivity (59.7%) for rabies diagnosis [63]. Camels were the second most likely livestock after cattle to test positive for rabies in Mongolia from 1970 to 2005 [45]. Camels were the fourth (4.2%) mainly rabies tested positive animals during 2004–2018 in China [46]. In China, rabies infection in camels was reported [8]. According to the confirmed rabies cases in Saudi Arabia during 2010–2017 [15], Dogs and dromedary camels were the most affected species. In Iran, a review on zoonotic diseases published articles [11] revealed that camels are one of the essential sources as well as carriers of infection for humans, livestock, and wildlife in Iran and worldwide. Rabies is highly endemic in Iran; it is circulated easily in wildlife and livestock. The authors reviewed reported camel rabies cases in Iran, 3 cases during 1996–2006; an outbreak of camel rabies was reported for the first time in 2008 in central Iran. A rabid wolf attacked 8 camels; another camel rabies in the east was reported in 2012 [11]. In Jordan, Rabies in 8 camels was described [12]. In India, a report of clinical signs of rabies in she-camel was described [4].

Reports of rabies in dromedary camels from Morocco, Mauritania, Sudan, Yemen, Saudi Arabia, UAE, Niger, Jordan, India, Israel, and Iran were reviewed by Abbas and Omer [19]. Ali et al. (2004) reviewed dromedary camel rabies in Sudan; the first confirmed rabies cases were in 1926, then laboratory-confirmed cases continued to be reported, 17 cases from 1927 to 1939, 21 from 1940 to 1970. Other cases were reported in different parts of the country, 21 in the north and 16 in the Western States. Camel population in Sudan is about 4.8 million; the reported rabies cases are very few compared to the population, which is mainly due to under-reporting. Other cases in camels were reported as well in Sudan [20].

In a review about camel diseases, many rabies cases have been reported in Mauritania, Saudi Arabia, Iran, and Pakistan; infection is usually due to rabid dog bites [68]. In Niger, an outbreak of rabies in the camel herd due to feral dog bites was reported [69].

Rabies outbreak in camels in Iran was described [70]. An outbreak of dog rabies in the camel herd was reported in Sudan in 1998, and it resulted in the death of 19 camels [71]. Antibodies against rabies were detected in non-vaccinated camels imported for slaughtering in Nigeria, which may indicate subclinical rabies infection [72]. Very few suspected rabies cases in camels were reported in Morocco during 1991–2015 [27].

8.2 Clinical signs

Camels with furious rabies form show restlessness, anxiety, salivation, and attacking and biting form followed by terminal paralysis, lateral recumbency (**Figure 6**) and a characteristic flexion of four limbs, reviewed by Abbas and Omer [19]. Mohammadpour et al. (2020) reviewed a report stating that a furious form of rabies is seen in most of cases in camels.

Rabies clinical signs observed in Bactrian camels were reduced appetite, excessive activity and agitation, cessation of rumination, lip twitching, hypersalivation, tachypnea and howling, paralysis [8]. Some reports described the occurrence of rabies dumb form more frequently. Most rabies cases (67%) in camels in Oman were

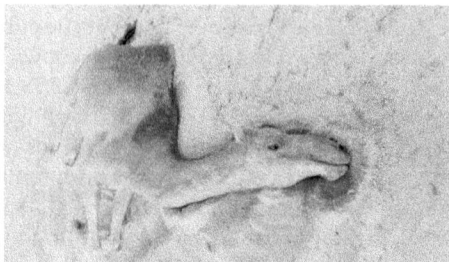

Figure 6.
A case of rabies in a dromedary camel showing lateral recumbency and excessive salivation.

of the dumb form; observed clinical signs were restlessness, salivation, head and neck rotation in all directions, paralysis, recumbency, and death [73]. Clinical signs seen in rabid camels were hyperesthesia, profuse salivation, anorexia, and paralysis [12]. In India, clinical signs of rabies in the camel described the appearance of hyperexcitability, bellowing, aimless running, salivation, convulsions, swaying of the hindquarters and recumbency, biting tendency to the owner and wooden objects [4]. Noticed rabies clinical signs in camels were unusual behavior including aggression, pica, ptyalism, and terminal paralysis [69]. During an outbreak of rabies in camels, reported clinical signs were high sensitivity, ferocity, biting faces of other camels, bloat, restlessness, limb paralysis, and yawning [70]. In a rabies outbreak, clinical signs noticed in most of the affected camels were restlessness, irritability with very harsh and loud sounds. Later excitement became noticeable. There were then rubbing incoordination (staggering gait), tenesmus, abnormal sexual behavior: (she-camels mounting each other), raising of tails, and slight salivation, terminated by paralysis of the hindquarter, recumbency, and death of 19 camels [71]. In Khartoum, two camel rabies cases in 1996, 1997 showed off food, salivation, nervous signs followed by biting fence and their forelimbs and abdomen, then recumbency, hind limbs paralysis, and death [74]. An almost similar picture was previously reported by Afzal et al. [75], which were hyper-excitability, salivation, attacking inanimate objects, biting of its forelimbs, sternal recumbency, paralysis of hind legs, and death.

8.3 Transmission

Transmission of rabies to camels is mainly through dog bites, except in some countries where wild animals like foxes and wolves are involved. In China, the main rabies transmitters are dogs; meanwhile, in border areas, the wild fox is [46]; camels were reported to be rabies-infected by dogs and wild foxes [8]. In Iran, a rabid wolf was reported to transmit the infection to camels [11]. In Oman, the main animals involved in rabies transmission are foxes [63]. In another study in Oman, it was noticed that most rabid camels were bitten by foxes, which confirmed the major role of foxes in rabies transmission [13]. In Saudi Arabia, the majority (70%) of camel rabies cases were due to wild dog bite, while wild foxes accounted for about 17% of cases [73]. Almost in all reported camel rabies cases in Sudan, dogs were the source of infection [18, 62, 71, 74]. The same finding was reported in other African as well as Asian countries, Niger [69], Mauritania, Saudi Arabia, Iran, and Pakistan [68], China [8] Saudi Arabia [15].

9. Rabies in pigs

9.1 Epidemiology

Pig rabies is not commonly reported; information about rabies in pigs is scarce. Tasiame et al. (2016) described an outbreak of dog-originated pig rabies in a herd of 23 pigs in Ghana with 13% mortality. In China, the first report for rabies cases in pigs was documented [7]. In China during 2011, an outbreak of pig rabies resulted in 14 deaths was reported [76]. In the USA, DuVernoy et al. [77], was the first to describe the clinical picture of a wild animal's originated pig rabies. During 2004–2018 in China, it was noticed that pigs were the least rabies-affected species (1.4%) compared to sheep, cattle, camels, and foxes [46]. In Brazil, Pessoa et al. (2011) reported the occurrence of pig rabies presented with neurological signs; it was attacked by a bat; there are several reports of detection of rabies virus in swine in Brazil. Preethi et al. (2020) reported the occurrence of pig rabies for the first time in South India; three pigs in a herd of 25 pigs were attacked by a stray dog. Osiyemi et al. [78] reported rabies cases in pigs in Nigeria.

9.2 Clinical signs

Observed clinical signs in pigs are anorexia, hyperexcitation, constipation, twitching of the head, and foaming [79]. Jiang et al. (2008) described clinical signs of rabies in pigs, the furious form was seen in almost all infected pigs, and it included hyperexcitation, roaring, and attacks on other pigs. In India, clinical signs in rabid pigs were aggressiveness, inability to stand with violent grunting, paralysis, lateral recumbency, convulsions, rapid chewing, head twitching, hyperexcitation, and profuse salivation, change in vocalization. Out of 25 pigs, mortality was 12% [5]. In the USA, rabies clinical signs that appeared in pigs were fever, restless-ness, salivation, aggression, anorexia, head rubbing, depression, vocalization, and progressive paralysis (DuVernoy et al., 2008). In Brazil, two pig rabies cases were reported: one with flaccid paralysis of the pelvic limbs; the other showed nervous signs, anorexia, and paresis, then pelvic limbs and tail paralysis. Generally, observed clinical signs were exclusive of the paralytic form [31].

9.3 Rabies transmission in pigs

Like other species, the transmission of rabies in pigs is mainly through dog bites and wild animals, especially in Latin America. In Brazil, Pessoa et al. (2011) reported the occurrence of bat-originated pig rabies. In the USA, DuVernoy et al. (2008) reported pig rabies caused by wild animals. In China, the first report for rabies cases in pigs was associated with dog bite [7]. In China during 2011, an outbreak of pig rabies was reported to be dog originated [76]. Tasiame et al. (2016) described an outbreak of dog-originated pig rabies in Ghana.

Acknowledgements

We are deeply indebted to Dr. Shamsaldeen Ibrahim Saeed for nicely drawing the illustrations (**Figures 1** and **2**).

Author details

Abdelmalik I. Khalafalla[1,2*] and Yahia H. Ali[3,4]

1 Department of Microbiology, Faculty of Veterinary Medicine, University of Khartoum, Sudan

2 Veterinary Laboratories Division, Abu Dhabi Agriculture and Food Safety Authority, Abu Dhabi, UAE

3 Department of Virology, Central Veterinary Research Laboratories, Khartoum, Sudan

4 Biology Department, Faculty of Science and Arts, Northern Border University, Kingdom of Saudi Arabia

*Address all correspondence to: abdelmalik.khalafalla@adafsa.gov.ae

IntechOpen

References

[1] CFSPH (2012). Rabies and Rabies-Related Lyssaviruses, CFSPH. Available at https://www.cfsph.iastate.edu/Factsheets/pdfs/rabies.pdf (accessed 22/04/2021)

[2] Uddin H., Nur-E-Azam M., Tasneem M., Bary M. A., Chowdhury P., Hoque M. A. (2015). Occurrence and management of suspected rabies in livestock species due to dog bites at Satkania Upazilla veterinary hospital, Bangladesh and Madras veterinary college hospital, India. Bangl. J. Vet. Med., 13 (2): 67-71 ISSN: 1729-7893 (Print), 2308-0922 (Online).

[3] Islam K.M.F., Hossain M.I., Jalal S., Kader M.N., Kumar S., Islam K., Shawn A.I., Hoque A. (2016). Investigation into dog bite in cattle, goats and dog at selected veterinary hospitals in Bangladesh and India. Journal of Advanced Veterinary and Animal Research, 3(3): 252-258.

[4] Kumar A., Jindal N. (1997). Rabies in a camel - A case report. Tropical animal health and production. 29. 34. 10.1007/BF02632346.

[5] Preethi D., Julie, B., Bhadra, P.V. (2020). Rabies in domestic pig- first report from South India. J. Indian Vet. Assoc. 18 (1): 123-127.

[6] Pushpakumara D.P.N., Ashoka D., Ranjani H., Preeni A., Craig S. (2019). Surveillance Opportunities and the Need for Intersectoral Collaboration on Rabies in Sri Lanka. Journal of Veterinary Medicine, Volume 2019, Article ID 7808517, 8 pages https://doi.org/10.1155/2019/7808517.

[7] Jiang, Y., Yu, X., Wang, L., Lu, Z., Liu, H., Xuan, H., Hu, Z., Tu, C (2008). An outbreak of pig rabies in Hunan province, China. Epidemiology and infection, 136 (04): 504-508.

[8] Liu Y, Zhang H-P, Zhang S-F, Wang J-X, Zhou H-N, Zhang F, et al. (2016) Rabies Outbreaks and Vaccination in Domestic Camels and Cattle in Northwest China. PLoS Negl Trop Dis 10(9): e0004890. doi: 10.1371/journal.pntd.0004890.

[9] Zhu Y., Zhang G., Shao M., Lei Y., Jiang Y., Tu C. (2011). An outbreak of sheep rabies in Shanxi province, China. Epidemiol. Infect, 139, 1453-1456.

[10] Simani S., Fayaz A., Rahimi P., Eslami N., Howeizi N., Biglari P. (2012). Six fatal cases of classical rabies virus without biting incidents, Iran 1990-2010. Journal of Clinical Virology 54: 251– 254.

[11] Mohammadpour R., Champour M., Tuteja F., Mostafavi E. (2020). Zoonotic implications of camel diseases in Iran Vet Med Sci., 6(3): 59-381.

[12] Al-Rawashdeh, O.F., Al-Ani, F.K., Sharif, L.A., Al-Qudah, K.M., Al-Hami, Y., Frank, N. (2000). A survey of camel (*Camelus dromedarius*) diseases in Jordan. Journal of Zoo and Wildlife Medicine 31(3): 335-338.

[13] Ahmed M. S., Body M.H., El-Neweshy M.S., ALrawahi A.H., Al-Abdawani M., Eltahir H.A., Mahir G. ALmaewaly M.G. (2020). Molecular characterization and diagnostic investigations of rabies encephalitis in camels (*Camelus dromedaries*) in Oman: a retrospective study. Trop Anim Health Prod, 52:2163-2168.

[14] Putra, K. S. A. (2018). Epidemiology of rabies. International Journal of Chemical & Material Sciences, 1(1), 14-24. https://doi.org/10.31295/ijcms.v1n1.4.

[15] Kasem S., Hussein R., Al-Doweriej A., Qasim I., Abu-Obeida A., Almulhim I.,

Alfarhan H., Hodhod A.A., Abel-latif M.A., Hashim O., Al-Mujalli D., AL-Sahaf A. (2019). Rabies among animals in Saudi Arabia. Journal of Infection and Public Health 12: 445-447.

[16] Omodo M., Gouilh M.A., Mwiine F.N., Okurut A.R.A., Nantima N., Namatovu A., Nakanjako M.F., Isingoma E., Arinaitwe E., Esau M., Kyazze S., Bahati M., Mayanja F., Bagonza P., Urri R.A., Lovincer M.N., Nabatta E., Kidega E., Ayebazibwe C., Nakanjako G., Sserugga J., Ndumu D.B, Mwebe R., Mugabi K., Gonzalez J. Sekamatte M. (2020). Rabies in Uganda: rabies knowledge, attitude and practice and molecular characterization of circulating virus strains. BMC Infectious Diseases (2020) 20:200 https://doi.org/10.1186/s12879-020-4934-y.

[17] Ali, Y.H; Intisar, K.S.; Wegdan, H.A.; Ali, E.B. (2006). Epidemiology of rabies in Sudan. JAVA. 5(3) 266-270.

[18] Baraa, A.M., Ali,Y.H, AbdelGadder Balal, Salma ElMagboul. (2012). Assessment of rabies situation in Sudan during 2007-2010. Sud J Vet Sci Anim Husb 51(1) 19-31.

[19] Abbas B., Omer O. (2005). Review of infectious diseases of the camel. Veterinary Bulletin, 75(8), 1-16.

[20] Ahmed B.A, Ali Y.H, Ahmed O., Elmagboul S, Ballal A. (2016). Detection of rabies in camel, goat and cattle in Sudan using Fluorescent antibody test (FAT) and Polymerase Chain Reaction (RT-PCR). Journal of Advanced Veterinary and Animal Research, 3(3): 274-277.

[21] Ali, Y.H. (2002). Outbreak of Rabies in south Darfur (Sudan). Vet Rec. 150 (19) 610-612.

[22] Nibret Moges N. (2015). Epidemiology, Prevention and Control Methods of Rabies in Domestic Animals: Review Article. European Journal of Biological Sciences 7 (2): 85-90, ISSN 2079-2085, DOI: 10.5829/idosi.ejbs.2015.7.02.93255.

[23] Reta, T., Teshale, S., Deressa, A., Mengistu, F., Sifer, D., Freuling, C.M. (2014). Rabies in animals and humans in and around Addis Ababa, the capital city of Ethiopia: A retrospective and questionnaire based study. Journal of Veterinary Medicine 6(6): 178 – 186.

[24] Oyda S., and Megersa B. (2017). A review of rabies in livestock and humans in Ethiopia. International Journal of Research - Granthaalayah, 5(6), 561-577. https://doi.org/10.5281/zenodo.823626.

[25] Mulugeta Y., Lombamo F., Alemu A., Bekele M., Assefa Z., Shibru E., Beyene M., kitila G., Getahun G., Sifer D., Aklilu M., Regassa F., Deressa A. (2020). Assessment of the current rabies situation and its management in epidemic areas of southern Ethiopia. Highlights in BioScience 3. Article ID 20212. dio:10.36462/H.BioSci.202 12

[26] Bitek A.O., Osoro E., Munyua P.M. Nanyingi M., Muthiani Y., Kiambi S., Muturi M., Mwatondo A., Muriithi R., Cleaveland S., Hampson K., Njenga M. K., Kitala P.M., Thumbi S.M. (2019). A hundred years of rabies in Kenya and the strategy for eliminating dog-mediated rabies by 2030 [version 2; peer review: 4 approved] AAS Open Research 2019, 1:23 https://doi.org/10.12688/aasopenres.12872.2.

[27] Darkaoui S., Cliquet F., Wasniewski M., Robardet E., Aboulfidaa N., Bouslikhane M. Fassi-Fihri O. (2017). A Century Spent Combating Rabies in Morocco (1911-2015): How Much Longer? Front. Vet. Sci. 4:78. doi: 10.3389/fvets.2017.00078.

[28] Ibrahim S, Audu SW, Usman A and Kaltugo BY (2017) Rabies in a Six-Week

Old Bunaji-Bull Calf in Zaria: A Case Report. J Microbes Microbio Techni 1(1): 101.

[29] Tekki I.S., Meseko C.A., Omotainse S.O., Atuman Y.J., Chukwukere, Olaleye S., Okewole P.A. (2014) Incidences of Rabies in Domestic Animals and Consequent Risk Factors in Humans. J Med Microb Diagn 3: 143. doi:10.4172/2161 0703.1000143.

[30] Suluku R., Nyandeboh J.P.J, Kallon M.N., Barrie A. Kabba B., Koroma B.M., Emikpe B.O. (2017). First Reported Case of Dog Associated Cattle Rabies in Koinadugu District, Northern Sierra Leone. Afr. J. Biomed. Res. 20 (3): 325- 327.

[31] Pessoa C.R.D., Maria Luana Cristiny Rodrigues Silva M.L.C.R., Gomes A.A.D., Garcia A.I.E., Ito F.H., Brandão P.E., Riet-Correa F.R. (2011). Paralytic rabies in swine. Brazilian Journal of Microbiology, 42: 298-302.

[32] Moreira IL., de Sousa., Ferreira-Junior JA., de CastroMB., Fino TCM., Borges JRJ., Soto-Blanco B., Câmara ACL (2018) Paralytic rabies in a goat. BMC Vet Res 14(1):338 doi: 10.1186/s12917-018-1681-z.

[33] Bárcenas-Reyes I., Nieves-Martínez D.P., Cuador-Gil J.Q., Loza-Rubio E., González Ruiz S., Cantó-Alarcón G.J., Milián-Suazo F. (2019). Spatiotemporal analysis of rabies in cattle in central Mexico. Geospatial Health, 14:805, 247-253.

[34] Gilbert A., Greenberg L., Moran D., Danilo Alvarez D., Alvarado M., Daniel L. Garcia D.L., Leonard Peruski L. (2015). Antibody response of cattle to vaccination with commercial modified live rabies vaccines in Guatemala. Preventive Veterinary Medicine, 118: 36-44.

[35] Botvinkin A., Kosenko M. (2015). Rabies in the European parts of Russia, Belarus and Ukrainea In Historical Perspective of Rabies in Europe and the Mediterranean Basin. Paris: OIE (World Organization for Animal Health) (2015). p. 47-63. Available from: http:// www.oie.int/doc/ged/d11246.pdf.

[36] Westerling B., Z. Andersons, J. Rimeicans, K. Lukauskas A. Dranseika. (2015). Rabies in the Baltics In Historical Perspective of Rabies in Europe and the Mediterranean Basin. Paris: OIE (World Organization for Animal Health) (2015). p. 33-46. Available from: http://www.oie.int/doc/ ged/d11246.pdf.

[37] Polupan I., Bezymennyi M., Gibaliuk Y., Drozhzhe Z., Rudoi O., Ukhovskyi V., Nedosekov V. De Nardi M. (2019). An Analysis of Rabies Incidence and Its Geographic Spread in the Buffer Area Among Orally Vaccinated Wildlife in Ukraine from 2012 to 2016. Front. Vet. Sci. 6:290. doi: 10.3389/fvets.2019.00290.

[38] Hampson K., Coudeville L., Lembo T., Sambo M., Kieffer A., Attlan M., Barrat J., Blanton J.D., Briggs D.J., Cleaveland S., Costa P.,Freuling C.M.,Hiby E. (2015). Estimating the global burden of endemic canine rabies. PLoS Negl Trop Dis (2015) 9(4):e0003786. doi:10.1371/ journal.pntd.0003786.

[39] Rinchen S., Tenzin T., Hall D., van der Meer F., Sharma B., Dukpa K., Cork S. (2019). A community based knowledge, attitude, and practice survey on rabies among cattle owners in selected areas of Bhutan. PLoS Negl Trop Dis 13(4): e0007305. https://doi. org/10.1371/journal.pntd.0007305.

[40] Samad MA (2013). Public health threat caused by zoonotic diseases in Bangladesh. Bangladesh Journal of Veterinary Medicine 9: 95-120.

[41] OIE, the World Organization for Animal Health (2018). Chapter 1.3.17.

Rabies (Infection with Rabies virus and other Lyssaviruses) (https://www.oie.int//fileadmin/Home/eng/Health_standards/tahm/3.01.17_ RABIES.pdf, accessed 11 March 2021)

[42] Reta, T., Teshale, S., Deressa, A., Getahun, G., Baumann, M.P.O., Muller, T., Freuling, C. M. (2013). Evaluation of rapid immunodiagnostic test for rabies diagnosis using clinical brain samples in Ethiopia. Journal of Veterinary Science and Medical Diagnosis 2(3):1-3.

[43] Bouaddi K., Bitar A., Bouslikhane M., Ferssiwi A., Fitani A., Mshelbwala P.P. (2020). Knowledge, Attitudes, and Practices Regarding Rabies in El Jadida Region, Morocco Khadija. Vet. Sci. 2020, 7, 29; doi:10.3390/vetsci7010029.

[44] Yahiaoui, Fatima & Kardjadj, Moustafa & Laidoudi, Younes & Hacene, Medkour, Ben-Mahdi, Meriem. (2018). The epidemiology of dog rabies in Algeria: Retrospective national study of dog rabies cases, determination of vaccination coverage and immune response evaluation of three commercial used vaccines. Preventive Veterinary Medicine. 158 10.1016/j. prevetmed.2018.07.011.

[45] Sack A., Daramragchaa U., Chuluunbaatar M., Battsetseg Gonchigoo B., Gray G.C. (2018) Potential risk factors for zoonotic disease transmission among Mongolian herder households caring for horses and camels. Pastoralism: Research, Policy and Practice 8:2. DOI 10.1186/s13570-017-0109-x.

[46] Feng Y., Wang Y., Xu W., Tu Z., Liu T., Huo M., Liu Y., Gong W., Zeng Z., Wang W., Wei Y., Tu C. (2020). Animal Rabies Surveillance, China, 2004-2018. Emerg Infect Dis. (12): 2825-2834. doi: 10.3201/eid2612.200303.

[47] Singh R., Singh K.P., Cherian S., Saminathan M., Kapoor S.,

Reddy M.G.B., Panda S., Dhama K. (2017) Rabies – epidemiology, pathogenesis, public health concerns and advances in diagnosis and control: a comprehensive review, Veterinary Quarterly, 37:1, 212-251, DOI: 10.1080/01652176.2017.1343516.

[48] Devleesschauwer B., Aryal A, Sharma B.K, Ale A., Declercq A, Depraz S., Gaire T.N., Gongal G., Surendra Karki S., Pandey B.D., Pun S.B., Duchateau L., Dorny P., Speybroeck N. (2016). Epidemiology, Impact and Control of Rabies in Nepal: A Systematic Review. PLoS Negl Trop Dis 10(2): e0004461.

[49] Taghreed A., Asmaa A. (2019). A Systematic Review of epidemiology of Rabies in Arab countries. Journal of Health Informatics in Developing Countries, 13 (2), http://www.jhidc.org/

[50] Hikufe E.H., Freuling C.M., Athingo R., Shilongo A., Ndevaetela E-E., Helao M., Shiindi M., Rainer Hassel R., Bishi A., Khaiseb S., Kabajani J, Westhuizen J. V., Torres G., Britton A., Letshwenyo M., Schwabenbauer K., Mettenleiter T.C., Denzin N., Amler S., Conraths F.J., Mu¨ller T., Maseke A. (2019). Ecology and epidemiology of rabies in humans, domestic animals and wildlife in Namibia, 2011 2017. PLoS Negl Trop Dis 13(4): e0007355. https://doi.org/10.1371/journal.pntd.0007355

[51] Van Sittert S. J., Raath J., Akol G.W., Miyen J.M., Mlahlwa B., Sabeta C. T. (2010) Rabies in the Eastern Cape Province of South Africa – where are we going wrong? Journal of the South African Veterinary Association 81(4): 207-215.

[52] Matter H, Blancou J, Benelmouffok A, Hammami S, Fassi-Fehri N (2015). Rabies in North Africa and Malta in Historical Perspective of Rabies in Europe and the Mediterranean Basin. Historical Perspective of Rabies

in Europe and the Mediterranean Basin. Paris: OIE (World Organization for Animal Health) (2015). p. 185-199. Available from: http://www.oie.int/doc/ged/d11246.pdf.

[53] Xiaoyue Ma., Benjamin P. M., Cleaton J. M., Orciari L.A., Yager P., Yu Li, Kirby J.D., Blanton J.D., Petersen B.W., Wallace R.M. (2018). Rabies surveillance in the United States during 2016. Journal of the American Veterinary Medical Association, 252 (8): 945-957.https://doi.org/10.2460/javma.252.8.945.

[54] Lima, E. F., Riet-Correa, F., Castro, R. S., de, Gomes, A. A. B., Lima, F. D. (2005). Sinais clínicos, distribuição das lesões no sistema nervoso e epidemiologia da raiva em herbívoros na região Nordeste do Brasil. *Pesquisa Veterinária Brasileira*, *25*(4), 250-264. https://doi.org/10.1590/S0100-736X2005000400011.

[55] Benavides J.A., Velasco-Villa A., Godino L.C., Satheshkumar P.S., Nino R., Rojas Paniagua E. R., Shiva C., Falcon N., Daniel G. Streicker D.G. (2020). Abortive vampire bat rabies infections in Peruvian peri domestic livestock. PLoS Negl Trop Dis 14(6): e0008194. https://doi.org/10.1371/journal.pntd.0008194.

[56] Acha PN (1981). A review of Rabies prevention and control in the Americas, 1970-1980. Overall status of Rabies. Bull. Off. int. Epiz., 1981, 93 (1-2), 9-52.

[57] Ahmad I., Kudi C.A., Anka M.S., Tekki I.S. (2017). First confirmation of rabies in Zamfara State, Nigeria—in a sheep. Trop Anim Health Prod, 49:659-662.

[58] Warrell M., (2010). Rabies and African bat lyssavirus encephalitis and its prevention, International Journal of Antimicrobial Agents, doi:10.1016/j.ijantimicag.2010.06.021.

[59] Chernet, A. and Nejash, A. (2016): Review of rabies control and prevention. Journal of Medicine, Physiology and Biophysics 23: 45 –53.

[60] Cifuentes J. J.F, Pérez L.R.D., Verjan G.N. (2017). Bat Reservoirs for Rabies Virus and Epidemiology of Rabies in Colombia: a review. Rev. CES Med. Vet. Zoot, 12 (2): 134-150.

[61] Ali, Y.H; Zeidan, M.I (1999) Rabies in Sudan 1992-1998: Sud. J. Vet. Sc Anim. Husb., 38(1,2)162-167.

[62] Ali, Y.H.; Intisar, K.S. (2009). Epidemiology of Rabies in Sudan (2003-2007). Sud J Vet Sci Anim Husb, 48(1,2) 104- 111.

[63] Al-Abaidani I.A., Al-Abri S.A., K.P. Prakash, M. H. Hussain, M. H. Hussain A.H. Al Rawahi. (2015). Epidemiology of rabies in Oman: a retrospective study (1991-2013). Eastern Mediterranean Health Journal, 21 (8): 591-597.

[64] Kaltungo B.Y., Audu S.W., Salisu, I., Okaiyeto S.O., Balarabe Magaji Jahun B.M. (2018). A case of rabies in a Kano brown doe. Clin Case Rep.; 6: 2140-2143.

[65] Tilahun A., Yohanis N., Biruhtesfa A. (2018). Review on Rabies and its Zoonotic Importance. Academic Journal of Animal Diseases 7(2): 29-38.

[66] Rissi, D.R., Pierezan, F., Kommers, G. D., Barros, C. S.L. (2008). Ocorrência de raiva em ovinos no Rio Grande do Sul. Pesquisa Veterinária Brasileira, 28(10), 495 500. https://doi.org/10.1590/S0100-736X2008001000009.

[67] Fowler, M.E (2010). Medicine and Surgery of Camelids. 3rd edition. Ames IA, Wiley-Blackwell.

[68] Fassi-Fehri M. (1987). Diseases of camels. Revue Scientifique Et Technique

(International Office of Epizootics), 6(2), 337-354.

[69] Bloch N, Diallo I. (1995). A probable outbreak of rabies in a group of camels in Niger. Vet Microbiol 46(1-3):281-283. doi: 10.1016/0378-1135(95)00092-o. PMID: 8545966.

[70] Esmaeili H., Ghasemi E., Ebrahimzadeh H. (2012). An outbreak of camel rabies in Iran. Journal of Camel Practice and Research, 19 (1):19-20.

[71] Elmardi O.I; and Ali Y.H. (2001) An outbreak of Rabies in camel (camelus Dromedaries) in North Kordofan state. Sud.J.Vet.Res. 17:125-127.

[72] Baba S.S., Bwala J.P., El-Yaguda A.D., Baba M.M. (2005). Serological Evidence of Rabies Virus Infection of Slaughter Camels (*Camelus dromedarius*) Imported To Nigeria. Tropical Veterinarian, 23 (3,4): 78-82.

[73] Al-Dubaib, MA (2007). Rabies in camels at Qassim region of central Saudi Arabia. Journal of Camel Practice and Research, 14: 101-103.

[74] Ali Y.H., Intisar K. Saeed, Zakia A (2004). Camel rabies in Sudan. Sud. J. Vet. Sci. Anim. Hus, 43(1,2) 231-234.

[75] Afzal M., Khan I. A., Salman R. (1993). Symptoms and clinical pathology of rabies in the camel. Vet. Rec., 133, 220.

[76] Yongwen L., Ying Z., Xiangyin L., Youtian Y., Xianfeng Y., Daiting Z., Xianbo D., Xiaowei W., Xiaofeng G. (2012). Complete Genome Sequence of a Highly Virulent Rabies Virus Isolated from a Rabid Pig in South China. Journal of Virology, 86 (22): 12454 12455.

[77] DuVernoy T.S. Mitchell K.C. Myers R.A. Walinski L. W. Tinsley M.O. (2008). The first laboratory-confirmed rabid pig in Maryland, 2003. Zoon. Pub. Health. 55, 431 435.

[78] Osiyemi, T.I., Onunkwo, O., Momoh, M.A. (1978). A case report of rabies in the pig in Nigeria. Bull Anim. Health. Prod. Afr. 26(4): 335-357.

[79] Tasiame W., Folitse R. D, Emikpe B.O, Adongo J. A. (2016). First reported case of dog associated pig rabies in Ghana. Afr. J. Infect. Dis. 10 (1): 55 – 57.

Chapter 6

Rabies Virus in Sierra Leone: Challenges and Recommended Solutions for Elimination by 2030

Roland Suluku, Emikpe Benjamin Obukowho, Abu Macavoray and Moinina Nelphson Kallon

Abstract

The objective of this write-up is to find possible solution control canine rabies virus in Sierra Leone and other low-income countries in the world. Rabies is a viral disease affecting both humans and animals in Sierra Leone. The country has no policy on dog ownership and management, two veterinarians, limited access to rabies vaccines and human immunoglobin, and a lack of information about the disease in the country despite increasing dog bite cases and death. There is no wildlife specialist to initiate wildlife vaccination. Continuous vaccination increased awareness, trained personnel in veterinary and wildlife, development of policies on responsible dog ownership and by-laws and increase financial support from the government and private sector will help Sierra Leone eliminate rabies in the first half of the twenty-first century.

Keywords: Rabies, Dog, Vaccination, Eradicate, Virus

1. Introduction

Rabies Virus is an acute, progressive, and fatal anthropozoonotic infection of the central nervous system belonging to the genus lyssavirus and family Rhabdoviridae that causes rabies [1]. History of rabies date back to work done by various con- tributors, such as Democritus (460–370 BC), Aristotle (384–322 BC), Pliny the Elder (23–79 AD), Galen (130–200 AD), Celsus (25 BC–50 AD), Rufus of Ephesus (80–150 AD), Oribasius (320–400 AD), and Aetius of Amida (502–575 AD) [2]. Records obtained from ancient Mesopotamian civilization approximately 4,000 years old associate rabies to bites by a mad or vicious dog [3, 4]. In the 16th century, Girolamo Fracastoro reported that when an animal bites and break into the skin it introduces the rabies virus [5]. In 1885, Louis Pasteur developed the first successful rabies vaccine [6]. Yet, rabies remains a threat to both humans and dogs in the 21st century [7, 8].

Rabies had been in Sierra Leone since antiquity but was isolated from the brain of the rabid dog at the Teko Central Veterinary Laboratory in Makeni, northern Sierra Leone in 1949 [9]. Rabies also existed in Kenema, Blama, and other parts of the country later found to be endemic with the virus.

Lack of veterinary staff prevented the government from developing poli- cies on dog ownership and management, undertaking large-scale research and awareness-raising on rabies [10] resulting in dogs receiving limited attention from their owners. Some could not feed their dogs, provide treatment nor pay for a rabies vaccine. With this obvious gap, rabies continues to take its toll on both humans and dogs. To combat this menace, the government focused on vaccinating dogs in major cities and outbreak communities providing high-cost rabies vaccines for affluent dog owners, while leaving dogs from low-income earners and the public unvaccinated. Liberia and other parts of sub-Saharan AFRICA reported a similar situation [11].

The death of thirteen people from 1968 to 1973 warranted government to vaccinate 4700 dogs in 1974 [12] which in turn gave prominence to control of rabies through a national vaccination of dogs which was short-lived due to the hosting of the Organization of African Unity (OAU) conference in the 1980s. The Government diverted meager resources to the hosting leaving most government departments unable to discharge their normal duties and service. Funding allocations to government departments dwindled and development in the veterinary sector diminished hence the inability to provide basic veterinary infrastructure and vaccination exercise for dogs and cats. No doubt, the difficulties, and hardship after the hosting of the OAU conference followed by political injustices brought resentment to governmental policies among the population.

Animal welfare occupied a lower primordial position on the list of national priority and family. This is also true across Africa where there is a lack of coordination and collaboration regarding dog ownership management, rabies control, and elimination activities, both within and across countries [12]. Most homes could no longer afford three meals a day and dogs have to cater for their daily survival. People focus their energies on their survival rather than dogs (Suluku et al. 2007). Dogs migrate with their owners during the war, which led to an increase in dog population in the capital city of Freetown and other district headquarter towns [13].

The bloody civil war (1991–2002) which brought untold suffering on the people of Sierra Leone was advantageous to dogs with many migrating to major cities and towns. The migration led to the increased urban population, congestion, and uncoordinated waste disposal in the city, the district headquarters towns, and refugee camps. In neighboring Liberia, the Lancet report 2014 reported a similar situation with a lack of electricity supply in large areas of the country especially after the rebel war from 1989 to 2003 and the devastating Ebola outbreak in 2014–2015. After the war, the crime rate increased and the need for dogs as guard dogs becomes inevitable for most people and families. Stray dogs do find food in garbage dumpsites, which enhanced survival and increased dog population, with a corresponding increase in dog bite cases. There is also no organized network of rabies actors to combat the escalating rabies cases in the country and at the regional level. However, some Africa regional groups such as Pan-African Rabies Control Network (PARACON) were established in 2015 to provide a forum to share information and provide available tools and knowledge to eliminate dog-mediated human rabies in Sub-Saharan Africa by 2030 [14].

2. Challenges of canine rabies virus control in Sierra Leone and other developing countries

2.1 Policies

Policies on dog ownership and management existed during the colonial era but were abandoned after independence. People and their dogs in the past received an annual rabies vaccine. The Government trained and empowered Police officers often called dog police, to impound, and penalized dogs' owners who failed to comply. The license and vaccination of dogs gradually disappear and dog owners no longer vaccinate their dogs against the rabies virus. Compounding the situation further is the complete lack of rabies vaccine in the country in the recent past and the prolonged civil war. Vaccinations of dogs are mostly done on an ad-hoc basis and only a few people especially children vaccinate their dogs. In most countries in Africa, people vaccinate their dogs on World Rabies day. Such spurious vaccination exercise will not eliminate rabies in the continent. The lack of effective policies on how people should own and manage dogs also tends to increase rabies outbreaks in the country. In China, for example, the national policy requires the availability of PPE (Personal protection equipment) in clinics in remote areas. Unfortunately, there was no information regarding the availability of PPE in remote communities in Sierra Leone [15]. Government across the African continent faces many challenges to effectively coordinate multifaceted programs of implementing the animal-human interface in the ecosystem in which they live [16]. The coordination of such structures is lacking in Africa and most countries have little or no public information concerning policies and strategies to eliminate rabies on the continent.

In the past decade, resource-poor countries in Africa are making some progress in rabies control and have increased their efforts due to a shift in policy by the tripartite group comprising FAO, WHO, and OIE to eliminate canine rabies by 2030 in African countries [17]. Despite this shift in policy towards canine rabies elimination, there is little public information concerning policies and strategies addressing canine rabies elimination for the whole continent.

2.2 Lack of veterinary personnel

Sierra Leone has only two veterinary officers employed by the government and three are lecturers at Njala University. The mandate of the Government veterinary doctors relates to the welfare of all animals in the country however, those deployed in the capital city are saddled with the administrative matter. With a higher rate of dog bites often reported every week by WHO, saddled administrative duties prevent them to do a follow-up on people bitten by dogs.

The lack of organized outreach programs by the government veterinary doctors and routine vaccination exercises for dogs make canine rabies control and elimination in Sierra Leone extremely difficult [18, 19]. This problem is not only affecting Sierra Leone but also other countries in sub-Saharan countries such as Angola, Botswana, Cameroon, Ethiopia, Kenya, Nigeria, Namibia, South Africa, Tanzania, Zambia, and Zimbabwe [20] where ethnoveterinary practices are commonly used to control of rabies.

2.3 Lack of information on rabies

The livestock division in the Ministry of Agriculture and Forestry from antiquity lacks veterinary personnel and other support staff to provide adequate information and services to animals and pets owners in the country. People do not know where to go when bitten by a rabid dog, nor is the vaccine available to treat both dogs and humans. Often human medical personnel refers dog bite victims to the veterinary doctor or clinics which implied that the knowledge of rabies and its treatment plan is low among medical personnel, especially in rural communities. The perception of the disease among the people is also poor as death associated with rabies is often attributed to witchcraft. Many countries in Africa have in one way or the order established a network to control rabies (40/54) however, there is still a lack of epidemiology data on rabies control and prevention [21] in both humans and other domestic animals [22]. In a review of dog control in West and Central Africa, it was reported that half of the countries in the two regions do not have reliable figures on dog population nor reported cases of rabies [23].

This obvious gap necessitates the need for research on the perception and knowledge of rural and urban dwellers on rabies and how best to handle dogs that bite people, this approach will help eradicate the disease in countries where 70% live in rural communities by 2030.

On the provision of vaccines, there is only one veterinary pharmacy located in the capital city of Freetown where animal owners and dog bite victims do patronize for rabies vaccines To increase awareness of rabies and the need for antirabies vaccination, the Animal Health Club initiated a rabies campaign between 2008 and 2013. With this effort, people became aware of rabies but lack vaccine to initiate large-scale vaccination exercises in the country hamper this laudable move to control the dreaded disease (Unpublished World rabies day report 2013).

2.4 Lack of wildlife specialist to engage in wildlife rabies vaccination

In Sierra Leone, the wildlife department in the Ministry of Agriculture and Forestry is responsible for all wildlife activities in the country. However, there had not been any anti-rabies campaign, especially for wildlife. Since the reservoirs of rabies are wildlife, vaccinating dogs against rabies without vaccinating wildlife is a fruitless endeavor, particularly when over 95% of dogs roam freely. This untamed or stray dog makes rabies eradication in Sierra Leone to be a herculean task to achieve by 2030. Currently, the wildlife unit is not adequately prepared for antirabies vaccination of the wildlife even though Njala university trains and graduates wildlife specialists every year.

2.5 Lack of follow-up on dog bite victims

After the establishment of the National Livestock and Animal Welfare Rabies Control Task Force (NLAWRCT) and the One Health Platform, the World Health Organization and the livestock officers, and community animal Health established animal bites (including dogs) surveillance across the country. WHO reports animal bites in a weekly meeting as shown in tables and figures 3.1, 3.2, and 3.3 respectively. Livestock officers including community animal health workers report to the Epidemiological unit in the ministry of agriculture which also share such information during weekly meetings with development partners but there was no strict follow-up by both partners and the government officers on the rabies status of the dog and the persons bitten by the dogs. The lack of reliable data on death due to rabies to inform government makes it impossible to allocate resources to rabies control. This pattern is consistent with most African countries where the level of the estimate of rabies burden is grossly lacking and insufficient to warrant investment [24].

3. Method to control and eliminate canine rabies by 2030

3.1 Formulation of by-laws

Since By-laws are rules or laws established by an organization or community to regulate itself, hence authorities and community members may establish and enforced by-laws to own and manage dogs [25]. Such acts and regulations should be enforced by the state veterinary services, and statutory animal welfare standing advisory committee should be in place to advise the government. These Established by-laws will help reduce rabies in communities, as was the case in the city of Craig in 1965.

In Sierra Leone, the Animal Health Club encouraged Villages around Njala University to formulate animal rearing by-laws. The club trained the villagers to wash and fed their dogs, the Animal Health Club provided groundnuts, seed rice, and cassava as an incentive for the children to care for their dogs in 2010. With this approach, communities have not reported any rabies incidents (Animal Health Club unpublished report 2010).

3.2 Responsible dog ownership

The concept of responsible dog ownership is a multifaceted social phenomenon intended to shape daily animal-human interaction [26]. Animals are increasingly becoming integrated into the human family in such a way that necessitates increasing attention and control [27]. It is therefore the moral responsibility of the owner to train the dogs in such a way that it conforms to the dictates of society. Dog owners are often to blame for the behavior of their dogs [28]. By providing sleeping places for dogs, feeding them at the appropriate time, providing water and treatment do make dogs behave responsibly, and reduce the chances of contracting rabies. Where such care is not in place, such dogs do scavenge for food in the nearest garbage, dumpsites, and neighborhoods. Such dogs around garbage dumpsites are often termed stray dogs, but most often are owned but unsupervised. Stray or unsupervised dogs often contract rabies through exposure to rabies virus from other street dogs and wildlife, which are a reservoir of rabies.

3.3 Continuous vaccination of both domestic and wildlife animals

Human beings have striven to eradicate pathogens of public health importance. Routine vaccination of diseases such as measles, polio, and diarrhea has saved over 10 million lives between 2010 and 2015 [29]. Successes of these magnitudes have convinced the World Health Organization (WHO), World Organization for Animal Health (OIE), the Food and Agricultural Organization (FAO) of the United Nations, and the Global Alliance for Rabies Control (GARC) to plan Canine rabies elimination by 2030. Their main elimination strategy is the continuous vaccination of both domestic dogs and wildlife animals. Domestic dogs present the greatest threat to public health particularly in poor countries where dog ownership and management policies are weak or non-existence such as Sierra Leone [30, 31].

Developed nations have successfully eliminated canine rabies through continuous vaccination of domestic dogs and wildlife, good dog ownership, and management followed by strongly enforced welfare policies [32].

In low-income countries including Sierra Leone, continuous vaccination of domestic dogs alone will not eliminate canine rabies because large-scale, dog vaccination campaigns should include vaccination of wildlife host species to effectively control or eliminate dog rabies [33]. Such a rabies vaccination campaign should utilize the One Health Approach to raise awareness. It should also be backed with strong bylaws, or animal welfare policies, effective dog population management, and strong political backing to eliminate canine rabies by 2030.

3.4 Training of canine and wildlife specialist in third-world countries

The reservoir of the rabies virus is mostly wildlife animals, but that which helps to transfer rabies to humans is a dog, 'man's best friend" Developing countries or low-income countries lack specialists in the area of canine and wildlife practice. In Sierra Leone and by extension West Africa need to train canine and wildlife specialists with a focus on rabies and other zoonotic disease control.

3.5 Development of the seven freedoms of animal welfare for developing countries

The five freedom of animal welfare originated from intensively kept animals often referred to as the golden standard developed by Professor Brambell and his team [34]. These five freedoms include Freedom from hunger and thirst, freedom from discomfort, freedom from pain, injury, and disease, Freedom to express normal and natural behavior, and Freedom from fear and distress. High-income countries like the United States of America, Europe, and South America have used this to eradicate and control the rabies virus.

The five freedoms do not apply to low-income countries where dogs scavenge in garbage dumpsites, feed through the hunting of rodents and wildlife animals they often roaming freely in the neighborhood and bushes during hunting.

Continuous vaccination of these dogs will not prevent rabies as they continuously interact with wildlife hence the need to complement the seven freedoms of animal welfare in low-income countries including Sierra Leone.

4. Tables and figures

The above data shows the number of and cats dog, cats bite cases, and people who have died of dogs and Cat bite cases in Sierra Leone from 2018 to 2020. The number of dog bite cases in 2018 was 1,354 cases resulting in 10 deaths while in 2019, the number of bite cases increased to 1, 544, but the number of death remains the same at 10. In 2020, 1,301 dog bites cases was resulting in 6 death. A personal interview with the Laboratory personnel of the National Central Veterinary Laboratory in Makeni reported that out of 10 dog bite cases reported about 90% are positive for rabies. Thus indicating the presence of rabies in the country. Out of 270 blood samples collected from dogs in the north, south, and east of the country, 24% show positive rabies antibodies in unvaccinated dogs (Unpublished PhD thesis, 2020). Sierra Leone is therefore far from rabies control if the above solutions are not properly taken into consideration (**Figures 1–3** and **Tables 1–3**).

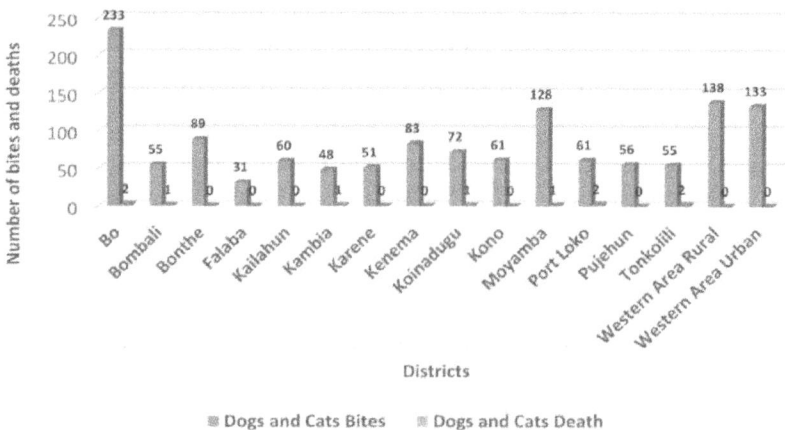

Figure 1.
Graph showing dogs, cats bites and deaths 2018.

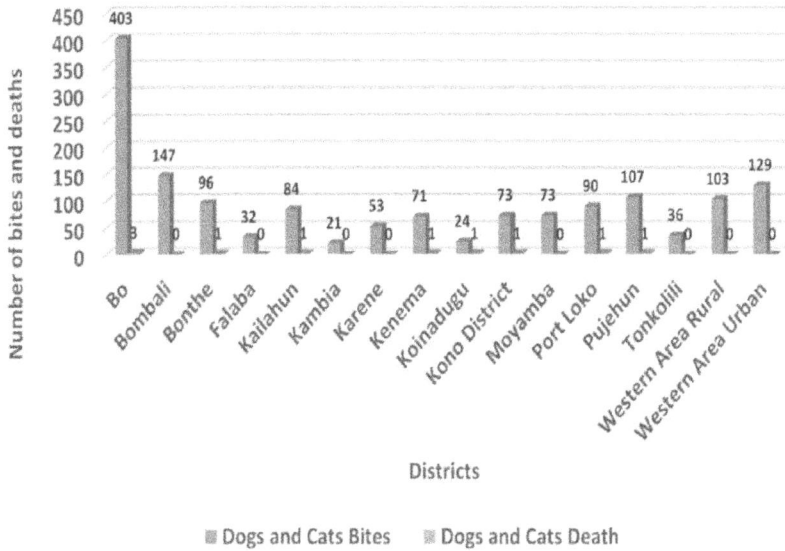

Figure 2.
Graph showing dogs, cats bites and deaths 2018.

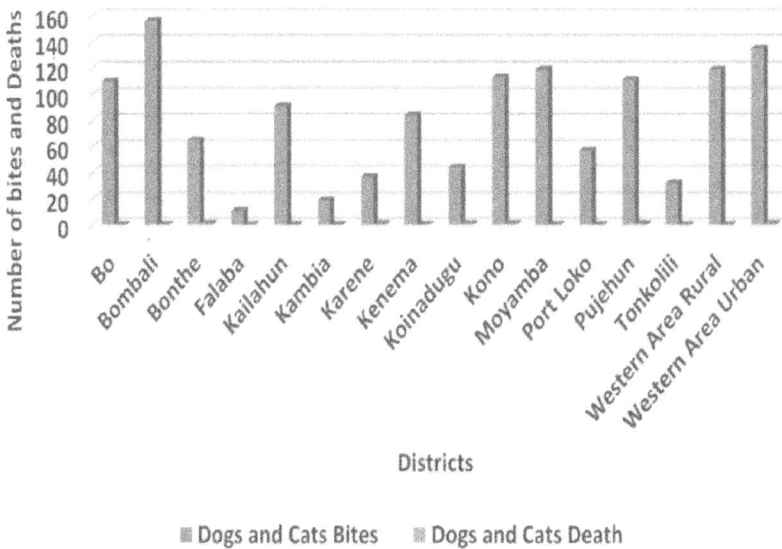

Figure 3.
Graph showing dogs, cats bites and deaths 2018.

Dog, Cats bites and Death 2018		
District	Dogs and Cats Bites	Dogs and Cats Death
Bo	233	2
Bombali	55	1
Bonthe	89	0

Dog, Cats bites and Death 2018		
District	Dogs and Cats Bites	Dogs and Cats Death
Bo	233	0
Bombali	55	1
Bonthe	89	0
Fallaba	31	0
Kailahun	60	0
Kambia	48	1
Kerena	51	0
Kenema	83	0
Koinadugu	72	1
Kono	61	0
Moyamba	128	1
Port Loko	61	2
Pujehun	56	0
Tonkolili	55	2
Western Area Rural	138	0
Western Area Rural	133	0

Source: Ministry of Health and Sanitation 2021.

Table 1.
Dog and cat bites and deaths 2018.

Dog, Cats bites and Death 2019		
District	Dogs and Cats Bites	Dogs and Cats Death
Bo	403	3
Bombali	147	0
Bonthe	98	1
Fallaba	32	0
Kailahun	84	1
Kambia	21	0
Kerena	53	0
Kenema	71	1
Koinadugu	24	1
Kono	73	1
Moyamba	73	0
Port Loko	90	1
Pujehun	107	1
Tonkolili	36	0
Western Area Rural	103	0
Western Area Urban	129	0

Source: Ministry of Health and Sanitation 2021.

Table 2.
Dog and cat bites and deaths 2019.

Dog, Cats bites and Death 2020		
District	Dogs and Cats Bites	Dogs and Cats Death
Bo	110	0
Bombali	156	0
Bonthe	65	1
Fallaba	11	0
Kailahun	91	0
Kambia	19	0
Kerena	37	1
Kenema	84	0
Koinadugu	44	1
Kono	113	1
Moyamba	119	0
Port Loko	57	0
Pujehun	111	1
Tonkolili	32	0
Western Area Rural	119	0
Western Area Urban	135	1
Source: Ministry of Health and Sanitation 2021.		

Table 3.
Dog and cat bites and deaths 2020.

5. Recommendations for the control of canine rabies in Sierra Leone

Rabies virus control in Sierra Leone and other developing countries requires awareness-raising using the Animal Health Club, One Health Strategy, vaccination of dogs (roaming and owned) and wildlife animals, formulation of by-laws for owning and managing dogs followed by the development of seven freedoms of animal welfare for developing countries.

a. Raise awareness using the Animal Health Club Strategy. Animal Health Club is an organization established to care for the health and well-being of both humans and animals (domestic and wildlife) living in a healthy environment. This club helps to raise awareness on diseases affecting both animals and humans using the One Health Approach [35]. In the case of the rabies virus, the club will work with the country's governance structure to raise awareness on the disease at the national, district, chiefdom, section, and town or village level. At National, the club contacts the appropriate ministries involved in rabies control, which include the Ministry of Agriculture, Health and Sanitation and Environment. Other Ministries include Education, Internal affairs, and Trade while the club will interact with Market women, traders, drivers, bike riders, Local artists, Paramount Chiefs, Town chiefs, and community elders (AHC Unpublished Report, 2012) to implement its activities on rabies and other zoonotic diseases.

At the district level, the club work with Directors, of the respective ministries to identify stakeholders involved in rabies and engages them in raising awareness on the disease at the district level. These involved District Medical officers, Agricultural Officers, Livestock officers, Health Education officers, environmental officers, Police Local Unit Commander and Military officers, Districts council officers, Mayors of cities. Principals and Head Teachers of secondary and primary schools, University lecturers and students, Local artists, Drivers' union, bike riders (often called OKADA), Petty traders, market women, and village town criers. Quiz, Drama, and debate competitions should be organized in schools, while local artists compose songs and act plays in their local dialects and 'Okada' or motorcycle riders drop rabies flyers, leaflets, and blow their horns to draw the attention of the public.

The club uses these and other media to raise awareness and sensitize people on rabies. Other media include Radio discussion and Phone-In programs, Jingles, distribution of flyers, handbills, and posters, composing songs in local dialects. Important personalities in the communities will commence the vaccination exercise as a show of commitment by the government, and other dignitaries in society.

b. Formulate dog ownership and management by-laws. The Animal Health Club engages the community, towns, or villages in a focus group discussion to understand challenges and constraints in owning and managing dogs, the consequences of rabies on dogs, people, and the community. Animal Health Club members help to edit the by-laws in simple English and read to the entire community, town, or village. Accepted by-laws are reprinted and distributed in Churches, mosques, schools and read to the audience. If the authorities did not receive any complaint, the by-law becomes binding. This approach was adopted in Njala University and surrounding communities to control rabies.

c. Conduct regular vaccinations of owned and unsupervised dogs. Such regular vaccination will drastically eliminate canine rabies in the community. Although sylvatic rabies exists in Sierra Leone, the continuous vaccination exercise in developing countries will contain the virus to a low ebb in low-income countries such as Sierra Leone. Vaccination of over 70% of dogs confers immunity against rabies in a community [36]. This statement holds for communities where they vaccinate both roaming and owned dogs and responsible pet ownership is strongly observed. However, if these dogs interact with animals in the wild, they are likely to contract rabies. These explain why rabies had not been successfully controlling or eliminate in these communities.

d. Established rehoming centers for unowned/unsupervised dogs.

In Sierra Leone, most people in rural communities do exchange items such as rice, chicken, ducks, and farm labor to obtain a dog. To reduce the stray dog population, there is a need to establish a rehoming center that will help to redistribute captured stray and unsupervised healthy dogs to communities and homes that desire to care for dogs. In this center, stray dogs that are terminally ill can be euthanized while healthy stray dogs can be treated, fed, and distributed to communities or people that desire to own dogs. Rehoming is a good strategy to control the stray dog population and reduce canine rabies infection. Sierra Leone has not established rehoming center, but plans are underway to establish such by the one-health platform. The rehoming centers also train new dog owners on how to cater to dogs.

e. Training of para vets or veterinarians to provide services to dog owners in countries where such personnel and veterinary services are limited such as Liberia, Sierra Leone, and The Gambia.

6. Conclusion

Rabies disease elimination requires concerted effort to control especially in low-income countries. The efforts should include the availability of the antirabies vaccine, sound policies on rabies virus control, a sufficient number of veterinary personnel, wildlife specialists, and adequate information on rabies with follow-up on dog bites. Adopting the Animal health club model, Formulation of animal rearing by-laws, enforcing responsible dog ownership, continuous vaccination of stray and owned dogs and wildlife animals, training of wildlife specialists and veterinarians with the development of the seven freedoms of animal welfare will help eradicate canine rabies virus in low-income countries including Sierra Leone before 2030.

Acknowledgements

The author wishes to thank the Ministry of Health for providing the data on dog and cat bites and members of the One Health platform in Sierra Leone and the Epi unit of the Ministry of Agriculture and Forestry for their valuable contributions. Special thanks to the staff of the Njala university One Health Serology and Molecular Diagnostics laboratory for the support.

Conflict of interest

The authors declare no conflict of interest

Research interest

Control of Zoonotic disease in rural communities through awareness-raising using the One Health Approach.

Author details

Roland Suluku[1*], Emikpe Benjamin Obukowho[2], Abu Macavoray[1]
and Moinina Nelphson Kallon[1]

1 Njala University, Freetown, Sierra Leone

2 University of Ibadan, Ibadan, Nigeria

*Address all correspondence to: nyasulukuroland2710@gmail.com

IntechOpen

References

[1] Leroy M, Pire G, Baise E, Desmecht D. Expression of the interferon-alpha/beta-inducible bovine Mx1 dynamin interferes with the replication of rabies virus. Neurobiol Dis. 2006;21(3):515-521. doi: 10.1016/j.nbd.2005.08.015. [PubMed] [CrossRef] [Google Scholar]

[2] Safari, B., Esnaashary, M.H. & Yarmohammadi, H. Rabies in medieval Persian literature – the Canon of Avicenna (980-1037 AD). Infect Dis Poverty 3, 7 (2014). https://doi.org/10.1186/2049-9957-3-7

[3] Rosner F: Rabies in the Talmud. Med Hist 1974, 18(2):198-200.

[4] Fekadu M: Pathogenesis of rabies virus infection in dogs. Rev Infect Dis 1988, 10(Suppl 4): S678–S683.

[5] Brightman C: Rabies: an acute viral infection. Trends in Urology & Men's Health 2012, 3(3):31-33. 16.

[6] Pearce JM: Louis Pasteur and rabies: a brief note. J Neurol Neurosurg Psychiatry 2002, 73(1):82 stoped

[7] Nadin-Davis SA, Fehlner-Gardiner C. Lyssaviruses: current trends. Adv Virus Res. 2008;71:207-250. [PMC free article] [PubMed] [Google Scholar]

[8] Woldehiwet Z. Clinical laboratory advances in the detection of rabies virus. Clin Chim Acta. 2005;351(1-2):49-63. [PubMed] [Google Scholar]

[9] Ministry of Agriculture and Natural Resources annual report

[10] Hikufe, E.H.; Freuling, C.M.; Athingo, R.; Shilongo, A.; Ndevaetela, E.-E.; Helao, M.; Shiindi, M.; Hassel, R.; Bishi, A.; Kaiser, S.; et al. Ecology and epidemiology of rabies in humans, domestic animals, and wildlife in Namibia, 2011-2017. PLoS Negl.

Trop. Dis. 2019, 13, e0007355. [Google Scholar] [CrossRef] [PubMed]

[11] Rabies control in Liberia: Joint efforts towards zero by 30Garmie VoupawoeaqrRolandVarkpehbVarney KamaraaSonponSiehcAbdallah TraorédCristianDe Battistie Angélique AngoteLuis Filipe L de JLoureirof BabaSoumarégGwenaëlleDauphinh WoldeAbebeiAndréCoetzerjk TerenceScottjkLouisNeljlJesse BlantonmLaurentDacheuxnSimon BonasnHervéBourhyn...Stephanie Mautinqr. (2021) Rabies Control In Liberia: Joint Efforts Towards Zero by 30. Acta.TropicaVol 216, April 2021. 105787. ScienceDirect ELSERVIER

[12] Andrea Haekyung Haselbeck,1,* Sylvie Rietmann,1 Birkneh Tilahun Tadesse,1 Kerstin Kling,2 Maria Elena Kaschubat-Dieudonné,3 Florian Marks,1,4,5 Wibke Wetzker,6 and Christa Thöne-Reineke. (2021) Challenges to the Fight against Rabies— The Landscape of Policy and Prevention Strategies in Africa. Journal List Int J Environ Res Public Health v.18(4); 2021 Feb doi: 10.3390/ijerph18041736 PMCID: PMC7916782 PMID: 3357904

[13] Ministry of Agriculture and Natural Resources MANR, 1967-1974),

[14] T.P. Scott, A. Coetzer, K. de Balogh, N. Wright, L.H. NelThe Pan-African Rabies Control Network (PARACON): a unified approach to eliminating canine rabies in Africa Antiviral Res., 124 (2015), pp. 93-100,10.1016/j.antiviral.2015.10.002

[15] Roland Suluku [1] Ibrahim Abu-Bakarr [2]Jonathan Johnny [2]F. Jonsyn-Ellis [3] (2012) Post-War Demographic and Ecological Survey Of Dog Populations And Their Human Relationships In Sierra Leone. (A Case Study Of Urban Freetown) Science Journal of Agricultural Research & Management

ISSN:2276-8572 http://www.sjpub.org/
sjarm-282.pdf. Volume 2012, Article
IDsjarm-282,7 pages,2012.doi:10.7237/
sjarm/282.

[16] National Health and Family
Planning Commission: Rabies Post-
Exposure Treatment Standard. [http://
www.moh.gov.cn/mohbgt/
s10695/200912/45090.shtml]

[17] Sinclair, J.R. Importance of a One
Health approach in advancing global
health security and the Sustainable
Development Goals. Rev. Sci. Tech. Int.
Off. Epizootic. 2019, 38, 145-154.
[CrossRef] [PubMed]

[18] WHO. Call to Tackle Rabies
Through One Health Interventions.
(2018) Available online at: http://www.
fao.org/ethiopia/news/detail-events/
en/c/1129639/ (accessed July 1, 2021)

[19] (PDF) Policy Perspectives of
Dog-Mediated Rabies Control in
Resource-Limited Countries: The
Ethiopian Situation. Available from:
https://www.researchgate.net/
publication/344080820_Policy_
Perspectives_of_Dog-Mediated_Rabies_
Control_in_Resource-Limited_
Countries_The_Ethiopian_Situation
[accessed Jul 01 2021].

[20] McGaw, L.J.; Eloff, J.N. Methods for
evaluating the efficacy of
ethnoveterinary medicinal plants.
Ethnovet. Bot. Med. Herb. Med. Anim.
Health 2010, 1-24.

[21] Eiki, N.; Sebola, N.A.; Sakong,
B.M.; Mabelebele, M. Review on
Ethnoveterinary Practices in Sub-
Saharan Africa. Vet. Sci. 2021, 8, 99.
https://doi.org/10.3390/ vetsci8060099

[22] Paulos. Y, Y.Eshetu, N.Bethlehem,
B.Abebe, Z.Badeg and B.Mekero,2003.A
study of Prevalence of Animal Rabies In
Addis Ababa During 1992-n2002.
Ethiopian Veterinary Journal 7:69-76.

[23] Céline .M et al,2020A Review of
Dog Rabies Control in West and
Central Africa

[24] Nel, L.H., 2013. Discrepancies in
data reporting for rabies, Africa. Emerg.
Infect. Dis. 19, 529-533, http://dx.doi.
org/10.3201/eid1904.120185.

[25] Haselbeck, A.H.; Rietmann, S.;
Tadesse, B.T.; Kling, K.; Kaschubat-
Dieudonné, M.E.; Marks, F.; Wetzker,
W.; Thöne-Reineke, C. Challenges to the
Fight against Rabies—The Landscape of
Policy and Prevention Strategies in
Africa. Int. J. Environ. Res. Public
Health 2021, 18, 1736. https://doi.
org/10.3390/ ijerph18041736

[26] Roland Suluku "Dogs of War"
Animal Health Club Champions Rabies
Prevention to Protect Livelihoods and
Lives in Sierra Leone published (2010).
FAO Agriculture and Consumer
Protection Department. Updated 25th
September 2012. Retrieved from www.
fao.org/ag/againfo/home/en/news_
archive/AGA_in_action/2010_Animal_
Health_Clubs.html.Journal of Animal
Production and Health Division FAO.

[27] Report of the Technical Committee
to Enquire into the Welfare of Animals
kept under Intensive Livestock
Husbandry Systems Chairman:
Professor F. W. Rogers Brambell, F.R.S.
Presented to Parliament by the Secretary
of State for Scotland and the Minister of
Agriculture, Fisheries, and Food by
Command of Her Majesty
December 1965

[28] Carri Westgarth, Robert M Christley,
Garry Marvin & Elizabeth Perkins
(2019) The Responsible Dog Owner: The
Construction of Responsibility,
Anthrozoös, 32:5, 631-646, DOI:
10.1080/08927936.2019.1645506 To link
to this article: https://doi.org/10.1080/08
927936.2019.1645506

[29] World Health Organization. WHO
expert consultation on rabies: second

report, world health organ Tech RepSer.2013;982:1-130. PubMed.

[30] Brown.K&Dilley.R(2012) Ways of knowing for 'Response ability' In more-than-human encounters: The role of anticipatory knowledge in outdoor access with dogs. Area,44(1),37-45

[31] Fox. R &Gee. N.R (2019) Great Expectations: Changing Social Spatial and emotional understandings of the Companion Animal-Human relationship. Social and Cultural Geography 20(1),43-63.

[32] World Health Organization (2017). Ten years of Public Health 2007-2017. Report by Margaret Chan, Director-General World Health Organization.

[33] Nelson. A (2016) Bringing the beast back in: The rehabilitation of pets keeping in Soviet Russia. In M.P. Pregowski(Ed). Companion animal in everyday life; Situating Human-animal engagement within cultures(pp43-580New York, NY Palgrave/Macmillan

[34] Fooks AR, Banyard AC, Horton DL, Johnson,2014: N, McElhinney LM, Jackson AC. Current status of rabies and prospects for elimination. Lancet;2014; 1389-99.DOI PubMed

[35] Velasco-Villa A, Escobar LE, Sanchez A, Shi M, Streicker DG, Gallardo-Romero NF, et al Successful strategies implemented towards the elimination of Canine rabies in western Hemisphere. A Res. 2017;143;1-12. Dol Pub Medntiviral

[36] Lembo T, Hampson K, Kaare MT, Enerst E, Knobel D, et al (2010). The Feasibility of Eliminating canine rabies in Africa Disspell doubt with data. PLoS Neglected Tropical Disease 4 View Article Google Scholar

www.ingramcontent.com/pod-product-compliance
Lightning Source LLC
Chambersburg PA
CBHW081235190326
41458CB00016B/5791